Professional Perspectives On Addiction Medicine

Volume 1

*Understanding Opioid Addiction and the
Function of Methadone Treatment*

Edited by

Mark Stanford, Ph.D.
Donald Avoy, M.D.

Professional Perspectives On Addiction Medicine: Volume 1
Understanding Opioid Addiction and the Function of Methadone Treatment

To those individuals who triumphed over their opioid addiction and are now living examples to others, we dedicate this work.

CONTENTS

Foreword

It's not difficult to obtain a variety of opinions about methadone, and chances are that should you do so, many of them would be quite negative and unfounded. This would be true if you were to ask people who have had no experience with this substance either directly or indirectly. Chances are, the person asked would not know anyone receiving methadone treatment, nor even know about someone receiving this treatment.

If you were to ask the opinion of several physicians, it is likely that you would again hear negative opinions, such as "that stuff doesn't work," or "that stuff is no better than heroin." And yet if you pursued the point and asked further questions, it would be likely that the physicians had never received any training in addiction treatment, and had never encountered a patient being treated with methadone for opioid addiction. The same might be the case if you asked many lawyers, or judges about methadone. You would find that not many knew much about it, but that the impression is generally negative.

Even within the areas of the addiction recovery community does there exist negative opinion about methadone treatment that can also stigmatize the methadone patient. There are still recovery communities that continue to believe that a person "can't really be in recovery from addiction if they are on methadone".

This in spite of the fact that methadone is widely accepted within the addiction treatment community as the most effective treatment for heroin addiction, has the best treatment outcomes compared to other modalities and is extremely effective in the prevention of HIV/AIDS and other diseases. This in spite of the fact that methadone dramatically reduces, and often eliminates, criminal activity. This despite the remarkable safety record of methadone after forty years during which it has been taken daily by hundreds of thousands of patients.

This pervasive lack of understanding is frustrating to those of us who see the other side of methadone, and are frustrated not only by the lack of understanding, but more by the stigma that has to be endured by those whose lives have dramatically benefited from it.

So we have attempted to take that frustration and convert it into a collection of presentations that will permit you to see methadone treatment through the eyes of a group of people who are involved in providing such treatment and are convinced that it has an important role to play in helping heroin-addicted patients recover control over their lives.

It is our hope that anyone who reads through this book will gain an increased awareness about methadone treatment, its foundation in evidence-based science and its effectiveness in treating opioid addiction within a variety of patient populations.

Donald R. Avoy, M.D.
Mark Stanford, Ph.D.

Introduction

Robert Garner

There is a well-founded science-base for understanding addiction as a chronic, and for many, recurring disease characterized by compulsive drug seeking and use. An abundance of research has consistently shown that chronic drug use affects the brain in fundamental ways often remaining long after the drug using behavior has stopped. Research science has also increased our understanding about the very nature of drug addiction, which has created new inroads for dramatic improvement in treatment approaches.

Using brain-imaging technologies, science can demonstrate the biological basis for addiction and has provided the basis for a biopsychosocial perspective of chemical dependency. From this knowledge we are now able to accept that for some addicted persons, medications are critical to treat drug-induced brain deficits in order to help sustain a symptoms-free lifestyle.

In much the same way that research provided for medications development used for other chronic diseases, such as hypertension, diabetes, and asthma, addiction medicine is following the same course.

Prior to the later 20th century, the general viewpoint of addiction, and particularly for opioid addiction, was that of a social and moral problem rather than a medical condition requiring treatment. The passage of the Harrison Narcotics Act in the early part of the 20th century also tended to stigmatize those with an opioid addiction reinforcing the perception that these people were not only as social deviants, but also criminals whose behavior deserved punishment.

Toward the latter part of the 20th century however, there was a growing change in the public's understanding and perception about addiction. Facilitating this change public perception was the introduction of the medical model of addiction as a treatable condition that helped to bring about an increase in human rights laws. Central to this was the introduction of methadone maintenance treatment.

The pioneering research by Drs. Dole and Nyswander began to reliably demonstrate that the medical use of methadone for the treatment of opiate addiction could significantly bring about normalization and functionality to those suffering from this condition.

Since then, research has continued to provide compelling evidence that methadone reduces, and often eliminates, criminal activity and at the same time, enhances social productivity. Numerous studies also have found that methadone is extremely effective in reducing/eliminating intravenous drug use and therefore also reduces the spread of infectious diseases including those such as HIV and hepatitis B and C.

Despite the volumes of independent research and scientific evidence from the last forty years about the safety and effectiveness of methadone for the treatment of opioid addiction, some of the social stigma and misconceptions about the medication have remained. Patients in maintenance programs are sometimes still perceived, even by health care professionals and parts of the recovery community, as "methadone addicts" who are simply substituting one addictive drug for another.

This book will put to rest any remaining doubt about the nature of opiate addiction being a chronic, reoccurring disease, and the value of methadone treatment for opiate addicts. And it should help end the unconscionable prejudice and discrimination that have faced opiate addicts for so long.

It is also intended to help the general public understand that persons addicted to opioids, much the same as victims of any chronic, relapsing disease, deserve to be treated with compassion and respect as they seek access to medical treatment for their disease.

We hope that the material will be used by policy makers in all fields that deal with opioid addicted clients, and by the various social service and health care systems who have opioid addicted clients in common where any misunderstandings about opioid addiction and the use of methadone as a treatment can be dispelled.

Chapter 1

Methadone Treatment - A Broad Perspective

Donald Avoy, M.D.

Introduction

Why would anyone want to learn about methadone? And, by the way, what is methadone? The word immediately conjures up dark images of depraved persons, perhaps fiends, receiving some dangerous material which they substitute for heroin. Professionals in the criminal justice system have viewed it with suspicion for forty years. It is poorly understood by most medical professionals. It is looked on with despair by the families of persons taking it. The general public is only vaguely acquainted with it.

This discussion is intended for persons in all the above categories in the hope that by better understanding addiction and its treatment, they will better understand the very important role methadone plays in the treatment of some kinds of addiction. Perhaps they might also have more understanding and compassion for those who are struggling with the formidable power of addiction.

Some Relevant History

Some archeologic remnants of poppy seeds suggest that this fascinating plant was valued by early members of our species, dating back to the end of the last ice age. But the first clear records we have were provided by the Sumerians, the people who inhabited the fertile valley between the Tigris and Euphrates rivers approximately 5000 years B.C.

The era in which our ancestors followed herds of animals on their annual migratory paths, sharing many of the same foods, gradually gave way to the time when they began to domesticate plants and animals and settle in one place rather than constantly moving. Fertile valleys would provide enough grain during the growing season to last the entire year. One of the other plants that was cultivated by the Sumerians was the poppy, which they called "the plant of joy"; more a testimonial than a description. The milky liquid that filled the seedpod was separated and dried. It could then be ingested --low and behold, powdered joy, now known as opium. We have no way of knowing how addictive this material was, nor how highly concentrated the active material was in the plants. . But we are able to know about the joyful plant because the Sumerians had developed a written language, which has provided descriptions of their culture.

After the two rivers meet in the middle of what used to be called Mesopotamia, they flow into the Persian Gulf, which provided the Sumerians an exit to lands and societies beyond. Overland, they could follow the upper reaches of the Euphrates through the upper arc of the "Fertile Crescent" and into the lands that bordered on the Mediterranean sea. These routes gave the Sumerians access to other societies, such as the Egyptians who began to enjoy the substance in about 2000 B.C. The Sumerians were succeeded by the Babylonians who carried the joy plant to Greece. We know that the plant was fondly regarded in Greece because it is described in Homer's Odyssey in about 1000 B.C. From there, Alexander the Great took it along with him when he invaded the Indian sub continent in 340 B.C.

The Romans used the poppy's power mostly for its calming, sedative properties. Hippocrates was an advocate of this approach. As trade developed with the Far East, the poppy plant extended its fame. In 400 A.D. it was being used in China for its anti-diarrheal effects.

Fast forwarding to the age of exploration, Europeans brought home the tobacco plant from the Americas along with the new technique of smoking. The Portuguese combined smoking and opium in the 16th Century and took both with them to India, where the new technique spurred greater production and use of the plant. When ingested with food, or in a beverage, as had been the method for many centuries, the onset of the effects of opium are somewhat slow, since the material has to pass through the digestive track before being absorbed into the blood, by which it can be carried to the brain. When smoked, the active materials get to the brain very quickly, within a few seconds, and the rapid increase in the concentration of that substance produces a more powerful, dramatic impact, which is now known as a "high", in contrast with the more mellow effect of ingested material. The practice of smoking opium rapidly spread through Persia and even to China.

In the 17th Century, an English apothecary, Thomas Sydenham combined the opium with sherry wine, producing a compound that became known as "Laudanum" which became a popular tonic for multiple and various ailments well into the 20th Century and gave rise to more opium addiction.

The growing power of the British Navy expanded the reach of the empire's economic force. The British East India Company, chartered by the crown, soon dominated the trade in opiates. The popularity in England of Chinese silks and porcelain made them eager to increase trade with China. The company began importing chests of opium into Canton, despite the prohibition of the Emperor. Canton was the only Chinese city in which the western ships were permitted to do business. Because it was located in the south of China, a long distance from the Emperor's palace in Peking, a robust smuggling business began to thrive.

Early in the 19th Century, a German chemist was able to extract the most active component from the juice of the poppy. He named the substance "Morphine" after the Greek god of sleep. Physicians began to focus on the two most powerful effects of this substance; it could bring sleep and it could relieve pain.

In 1843 a Scottish physician, Alexander Wood, developed a new technique for administering morphine with a syringe, which made the effects more immediate and more powerful. This immediately was put to use on the battlefield, first in the Crimean war in Russia and only slightly later in the American Civil War. With the new medicine, physicians were able to perform much more aggressive battlefield procedures, many of them amputations, to save the lives of the wounded. Many of those who survived the war and the surgery, later learned the cruel truth that they were addicted to morphine.

Back in China in 1848, when the Emperor learned of the smuggling of opium, he ordered the chests of opium to be seized and destroyed. With characteristic indignation, the British declared that this was the wanton destruction of the property of her Majesty, Queen Victoria, which provided the excuse to declare war. The frail Chinese ships were no match for the British warships. After a brief conflict, the British were able to impose new trade rules and open other Chinese ports to western trade.

When the Civil War ended in this country, the building of the transcontinental railroad began. Two companies were selected. The Union Pacific was to build west from Omaha, while the Southern Pacific built east from Oakland. It was a race because the companies were paid not only by the mile of track completed; they also received substantial land on both sides of the track. The Union Pacific speedily crossed the flat plains while the Southern Pacific was bogged down with labor problems and the menacing reality of the Sierra Nevada Mountains.

Unable to find sufficient, suitable labor, Charles Crocker, one of the "Big Four" owners of the Southern Pacific, reluctantly decided to try Chinese laborers. To his surprise, they proved to be strong, diligent and far more reliable than the Irishmen he had been using. In addition to their meager pay, they were given opium to smoke, which made them very tranquil, and reduced their libido and aggressiveness. They were able to toil through the winter snows working in snow sheds or galleries, constructed to protect the rails from winter avalanches, blasting tunnels through obdurate granite with the newly invented dynamite. Crocker imported thousands of Chinese workers for his railroad.

Meanwhile in the polite literate societies on both sides of the Atlantic, many famous authors were using opium to stimulate their muses. In Europe, these included Keats, Colleridge, Dickens and Browning. An Englishman named deQuincy wrote a memoir entitled "The Confessions of an Opium Eater", in which he graphically and enthusiastically described the effects of his habit. In America, Edgar Allen Poe, Walt Whitman and Jack London were among those who frequented the raptures of the poppy.

Late in the 19th Century, a most tragic irony took place. Chemists had discovered that by simple means they were able to convert morphine into another compound that they believed would be very effective in treating morphine addiction. They enthusiastically described how they had been able to substitute the new compound for the morphine and cure people of the terrible addiction. The Bayer Company in Germany began to market and supply this wonderful compound. They named it "heroin." Only after many people were so treated did they realize to their horror that heroin was more addictive than morphine. Bayer quickly took it off the market.

This incident and others brought the international community to focus on the perils of opiate addiction on a worldwide basis. The International Opium Commission met in Shanghai in 1909. The British were convinced to stop the opium traffic between India and China, to the relief of the Chinese. The international pressure led the U.S. to pass of the Harrison Narcotics act in 1914.

While the intent of this legislation was laudable and the wording benign, it was ultimately interpreted as banning physicians from treating addicts under penalty of losing their licenses to practice medicine. This led to the withdrawal of the medical profession from dealing with addiction and, by default, leaving it to the criminal justice sector.

During the 1930s, the U.S. Public Health Service opened three hospitals for addicted persons. These were primarily intended to serve as centers for treating addicted persons who had been incarcerated in federal prisons. However, some important experimental work was done which elucidated the predictable sequence and severity of withdrawal from opiates such as morphine and heroin. Attempts to prevent or alleviate such symptoms were less successful. Studies in the late '30s indicated that attempts at behavioral modification or psychotherapy were ineffective in having lasting benefit for addicted persons. The relapse rates were greater than ninety percent.

During World War II, Germany was cut off from its supply of opium, and therefore had inadequate supplies of morphine to treat battlefield injuries. German chemists were set to work to find a substitute for morphine and came up with a compound that was quite effective at relieving pain. That compound was methadone.

After the war, large amounts of opium began to be shipped from Turkey to Marseilles, where it was converted into heroin and smuggled into the U.S., mostly into New York. This was the now legendary "French Connection" which led to an alarming increase in heroin addiction, drug-related crime, fatal overdoses and other medical consequences.

An eminent endocrinologist with a brilliant record in research, but with no experience in addiction medicine, was asked to bring his scientific acumen to bear on the crisis. Vincent Dole accepted the challenge. Realizing how little he knew about the dynamics of addiction, he first studied volunteers who were heroin addicts. He brought them into the clinical research ward at the Rockefeller Institute and gave them heroin, as much as they wanted. He observed that they swung from being high to being sick from withdrawal several times a day, each cycle being terminated by another injection of heroin, subsiding withdrawal symptoms, and blissful repose.

Endocrinologists are experts at metabolism, i.e. the way in which the organism processes the chemicals that sustain life. Dole immediately postulated that the heroin was being rapidly removed from the body, leading to the withdrawal symptoms, which necessitated more heroin. One part of the solution, he believed, would be to find an opiate, which was removed more slowly. Another desirable characteristic of this substance would be that it should be effective orally, to avoid the medical consequences and dangers of injection.

He knew that scientists at the Lexington facility had attempted to substitute other opiates, including methadone, for heroin and had not been successful in halting the cycle of addiction. He decided to repeat the experiences using higher doses. He observed that when he substituted higher oral doses of methadone the wild swings between being high and being in withdrawals ceased. The patients began to behave more normally, and take interest in subjects unrelated to heroin use or its acquisition. He realized then that the addicts only needed a single dose every twenty-four hours, and postulated that this compound was metabolized dramatically more slowly than heroin, which was later proven correct when laboratory methods for assaying plasma methadone levels became available.

As their experience grew, Dole and his collaborators, Drs. Marie Nyswander and Mary Jane Kreek, became convinced that they had the right compound, methadone, which could be used to treat heroin addiction. They began to share their observations and results with the scientific community, and other investigators began to use methadone for their patients.

The criminal/justice sector was not enthusiastic. They considered it lunacy to provide opiates to persons with addiction to them. There were attempts made to close down the experiments and prevent others from continuing down this pathway. However, the Rockefeller Institute threw the full weight of its prestige and influence into the fray and the treatment advocates won the battle.

Based on the successes of Dole and his associates, methadone programs were started in Chicago by Dr. Jerome Jaffe and in

Washington D.C. by Dr. Robert DuPont which mirrored and validated the concept of outpatient treatment of heroin addiction with single dose, oral methadone.

Politics Meets Methadone

Early in the Nixon Administration, White House staffers were looking for new opportunities for political success. Some believed that drug treatment programs, then still in their infancy, might be such an opportunity. But this ran counter to the general orientation and convictions of the president. He was being hounded by anti-Vietnam War protesters; the same hirsute, promiscuous, drug users who would be the beneficiaries of a policy that was "soft" on drugs and drug users. That changed suddenly.

In April 1971, two congressmen visited our troops in Vietnam because they were alarmed by reports from their constituents that heroin abuse was rampant among the enlisted men stationed there. They returned with testimony that this was indeed the case. Later evidence indicated that as many as forty percent of the enlisted men had tried heroin and one half of them had become addicted.

This was a potential political bombshell. The war was extremely unpopular and evidence that the young people sent to fight were being subjected to a new menace would only add fuel to the fire. The spectre of returning veterans who would end up as addicts, involved in crime to support their habit, was horrifying. The Department of Defense had attempted to crack down on the problem but their only answer was to prosecute offenders, which was slow and ineffective as a deterrent.

The White House sent for Dr. Jaffe and asked him to evaluate the problem and suggest a program. He had recently learned of a new laboratory test that could detect heroin in the urine. This made it possible to screen large numbers of people. Jaffe urged that those ready for transfer home be required to provide urine specimens, and that those found to be using heroin be immediately placed in methadone treatment.

The plan was implemented and Dr. Jaffe was brought into the Nixon White House as the first in a long line of so called "Drug Czars". Nixon then announced that there would be a high priority given to stamping out drug abuse. The "War on Drugs" had been declared.

There were those in the criminal/justice sector that were aghast that the administration would embark on a program that seemed so antithetical to the expected "hard line on criminals" posture more characteristic of Nixon. They were mollified by being assured that the program would be carefully regulated and that they would play a large role in preventing it from getting out of control. In fact, methadone has been the most regulated drug in the formulary. Until very recently, there were several overlapping federal agencies regulating, licensing and inspecting methadone programs, in addition to state regulations. The regulations were very restrictive, including limiting doses in some cases. Recent improvements reflect the more appropriate attitude that these critical decisions should be made by physicians working on site, not by bureaucrats and politicians.

What Is Methadone?

In an earlier section, the ways in which different foods and other substances have been incorporated into primitive cultures have been described. This is an example of utilizing the native substance without any attempt to change it. Later, the chemical process of isolating the active ingredient, morphine, from the poppy juice was described. This would be termed a chemical extraction.

Still later, the processes by which codeine and heroin were obtained by chemically altering morphine were mentioned. These altered compounds would be called semi-synthetic. Methadone illustrates another process and a different final product, which is termed synthetic since it does not depend on the incorporation or alteration of a naturally occurring substance.

In the 1930s, one of the premier chemical companies in the world was the I.G Farben Corporation in Germany. Chemists employed by Farben were successful in producing compounds that were patented and controlled by the company. This was the same company that had been successful in producing heroin by altering morphine. The devastating reality that heroin was at least as addicting as morphine was a severe jolt to the company and set them onto a more difficult path. They began a project to find a compound that would be as effective as morphine for pain relief and not have the terrible price of addiction. (That search goes on today.)

In 1937 Drs. Max Eisleb and Gustav Schaumann came up with a novel compound, which is now known as pethidine. They could demonstrate that it did indeed have analgesic properties that were quite impressive. Alas, it also proved to be addictive. That compound is still used throughout the world, known in some countries still by the name of pethidine, in the United States it is better known as meperidine or Demerol. It is still used in obstetrics where it's brief duration of action is often valuable.

In 1938 Drs. Max Bockmuhl and Gustav Ehrhart announced that they believed they had solved the problem. Because the Farber plant was located at Hochst-am-Main, the serial number for the product was Hochst-10820 and the name they eventually used was Palamidon.

Because of the focus of the entire German nation on preparation and support for the war, there is a hiatus in our knowledge of exactly what happened during the next few years, but it is known that all the synthetic analgesics that were produced by Farben were used in place of morphine which was no longer available to the Germans.

When Germany collapsed in 1945, the Americans took control of the Farben plant and all its scientific and intellectual properties. These were acquired by Eli Lilly, the American pharmaceutical giant. That same year, the U.S. Department of Commerce published a report on a new compound, which had been renamed Methadone or Dolophin. While it could be demonstrated that methadone did have impressive analgesic properties, it's pharmacologic profile did not distinguish it from other competitors sufficiently to make it a clinical or commercial success.

It was, however, used in the research carried out in the U.S. Public Health's addiction treatment hospitals in which it was not particularly distinguished. The story might have ended there if it had not been for Dr. Vincent Dole and colleagues.

How Does Methadone Work?

The history of pharmacology is one of trial and error. Our ancestors used remedies that were passed on from generation to generation, usually herbs or roots that had proven to have therapeutic value over the years. Those that produced illness or death were considered to be the special plants of the gods who were angered when tried by mortals. Only in the last century have we learned that compounds which have the ability to produce significant changes in our bodies, do so, in many cases, because they attach themselves to chemical structures on the cells of our organs, called receptors.

Thus, the first mystery of why a plant like the foxglove can have dramatic benefit on the heart of person in congestive heart failure is solved. The flowers of the plant contain a chemical known as digitalis, which attaches to receptors on the cells of the heart muscle and makes the muscle fibers more efficient. Another mystery awaits; why would the heart muscle of homo sapiens have receptor for a substance found in a plant. We'll get to that later.

When the compound, the medicine, attaches to the receptor, on the surface of the cell, it causes the cell to go through biochemical changes. It may cause a cell in the adrenal gland to secrete adrenalin or adrenal steroids. It may cause the thyroid to produce more or less thyroid hormone.

When heroin, or morphine are eaten, smoked or injected, they are ultimately carried to the brain by the blood. In the brain, they attach to certain cells, in certain areas of the brain, that have specific structures, now named opiate receptors. These brain cells, called neurons, then release a chemical messenger or "neurotransmitter" called dopamine, which, in large amounts, can cause the rapturous experience known as the "high".

But there are opiate receptors in other organs in the body. For example, in the intestines, when opiates attach to the receptors, they slow down the intestine, which is why opiates have been used as treatment for diarrhea. In the lung there are sensors that detect the presence of minute particles that can cause damage to the delicate tissues. These sensors send signals to certain parts of the brain that initiate the cough reflex that expel the particles. Opiate receptors decrease the sensitivity of the neural network that leads to coughing, which is why opiates are used in upper respiratory infections to suppress cough. (Even though methadone does not have a plant origin, it attaches itself to the same opiate receptors.)

All organisms are in a constant state of renewal. Cells and tissues are constantly being removed and replaced. Small molecules, which are manufactured by the organism, are also chemically altered and excreted. The same is true for medicines, which is why one has to take many medicines on a regular schedule so the desired benefit won't wear off.

Heroin is removed from the body in a few hours. It is chemically altered by the liver to make it water soluble, and then is excreted by the kidneys in the urine. As a consequence, heroin addicts must "fix" three or four times a day. As was mentioned above, methadone is removed much more slowly, so that a single daily dose is usually sufficient to maintain a therapeutic level.

One of the most important functions of the brain is to maintain balance of all the chemical reactions that ultimately define life. Many of the reactions that are constantly taking place twenty-four hours a day, throughout our lives, are controlled by facilitators called enzymes, which are also chemical molecules. If the temperature of the organism rises, the enzymes work more rapidly, until at some temperature, the heat begins to disrupt the enzyme and it no longer functions. On the other hand, as the temperature cools, the speed of the reaction slows down, until at some temperature, it will cease.

The brain must monitor the body's temperature to maintain it within the range where the vital chemical reactions will continue. It must be able to lose heat when the internal temperature climbs, and it must conserve and generate heat when it falls. The same is true for acid-base balance, oxygen supply and a whole host of critical parameters that are the essence of life on our planet. Wide swings of these factors cannot be tolerated. They must be detected and adjusted back to within the life-sustaining limits.

When a large amount of heroin is injected into the blood stream, it stimulates a delicate system that has evolved to deal with gentle oscillations that might be compared to the ebb and flow of waves at the edge of a quiet sea. After the first injection, the system is suddenly engulfed by a virtual tsunami of chemical energy that is beyond anything previously experienced. So while the person is experiencing the high, the brain is frantically attempting to restore a balance that is compatible with continued life.

Moreover, it is also beginning to erect a chemical defense system that will prevent such a catastrophe in the future. The heroin is removed by the liver and kidneys and life goes on, but the brain is now more vigilant. On subsequent injections, the brain will oppose the effects of the heroin with a chemical counterbalance, so that the person will experience a diminished high. The usual pattern is that the person will find that they have to inject ever-increasing amounts of heroin and experience ever-decreasing rapture. This phenomenon is known as "tolerance," and it is common to all opiates.

But there is a more serious, ironic consequence to this battle between the brain and the injections. After the dose is injected, the process of metabolic transformation and elimination of the heroin begins. But the defense system has chemical "weight" that is balanced by the injected heroin. When the heroin is removed, that weight is unbalanced and it begins to produce the constellation of symptoms that are known as withdrawal symptoms, or "drug sickness."

The symptoms begin with vague uneasiness and irritability. But as the time from the last dose increases, they include sweating and chills, nausea and stomach cramps, which progress to nausea, vomiting and diarrhea; diffuse muscle and joint aches and pains. None of these is catastrophic by itself, but when the complete syndrome is established and getting progressively worse, it drives the person to seek relief in the form of another injection or dose of heroin which will quickly restore the balance and relieve the symptoms, making them feel more normal. As the months and years of addiction slide by in the twilight mental state of addiction, the person obtains less and less of the positive incentive of the high and more and more of the negative misery of withdrawal. And so ultimately, it is the brain's defense against the continuous onslaught that becomes the engine that drives the dynamics of addiction.

Methadone is effective because, after a single oral dose, it occupies the opiate receptors and prevents withdrawal symptoms. Further more, when an adequate dose is established, it prevents the craving for heroin that fuels the continuing compulsion to seek the drug.

Why Do We Have Opiate Receptors?

This question came up earlier, and it is a very important question. If evolution has selected for those characteristics that make it possible to survive on this planet, why would our genetic code provide for the synthesis of a structure that responds to interaction with a substance found in one particular plant?

In the early 1970s scientists discovered that there were specific sites in the brain of mammals that would bind morphine and other opiates that were labeled with radioactive markers, and that these sites were located in specific areas of the brain that were involved in the perception of pain. They began to postulate that these receptors were actually intended to be interacting with a substance produced by the animals themselves, and that the plant molecule was active because it was similar in molecular structure.

This led to a search for such a substance, and it was eventually located, purified, and the amino acid sequence identified. The substance was considered to be endogenous, that is, produced by the organism itself, and to have properties similar to m<u>orphine</u>. Thus, it was named endorphin. Since then, scientists have been working to define the functions of the endorphin molecules.

Even though the several compounds that have been found to be a part of the family of endorphins are quite small, only a approximately thirty amino acids in length, there has been a growing realization that they play a very important part in enabling our species to successfully inhabit this planet. If a species is to survive, there are certain functions that it must continue to perform, such as eating and procreation. If these functions result in a positive experience, it will benefit not only the individual organism, but also the species as a whole.

On the other hand, survival also entails avoiding those phenomena that are likely to impair the ability to successfully remain on the planet eating and procreating. Pain, or more accurately, the anticipation of pain, is a very powerful signal which will cause the organism to avoid being damaged or destroyed. From the discussions above, it is clear that the opiate receptors, and the endorphins are critical components of the neurologic systems that deal with pain and pleasure, so critical to our survival.

Beyond the more mundane pleasures of eating, are the responses to certain experiences and events that can better described as evoking a thrill; a rapturous sense of well being, accompanied by physical sensations such as gooseflesh, or a sudden chill. These can be evoked by a beautiful sunrise or sunset, the first cries of a new-born offspring, the sound of certain music, standing in the Sistine Chapel and seeing Michaelangelo's frescoes. These "epiphanies" are the jewels in the crown of our existence, and at the center of them is the neurobiologic network that includes the opiate receptors and the endorphins.

These fascinating molecules have been associated with an impressive array of human functions, and from this we may infer that they play similar roles in all vertebrates. Heavy exercise will increase the endorphin level, which produces the "runners high". Certain foods, including chocolate increase endorphins. It is now believed that acupuncture relieves pain by releasing endorphins. Changes in mood can involve endorphins. They appear to be released in response to prolonged laughter. There also appears to be a link between endorphins and the immune response. It's a very impressive list that involves a lot of the ways in which we experience the qualitative dimension of our lives on this planet. The endorphins are also involved in the body's response to stress, which will be discussed later.

Relapse--A Central Problem

When the Public Health Service began to study addiction, they brought volunteers to their isolated clinics who went through intensive rehabilitation. Even though they were abstinent for considerable intervals, when they returned to more natural environments, they almost always relapsed

Over the years, it has become clear that injecting heroin multiple times per day for years or even decades produces profound, durable changes in the neurochemistry and probably in the neuroanatomy of addicted persons. It is not uncommon for such persons to be able to have periods of abstinence, terminated by a relapse to heavy drug use, which produces profound shame, humiliation and even depression. Addiction is currently understood as a chronic, relapsing disease of the central nervous system and must be approached accordingly, which means that superficial slogans or magical cures are extremely unlikely to be effective.

Why do people relapse? The answer is that even though they have been abstinent, the neurobiologic changes inflicted on their brains by long term addiction have not been returned to normal, and they are therefore, still vulnerable to certain stimuli, called "triggers". Examples of triggers include, exposure to the substance or paraphernalia of their addiction, i.e. just seeing a heroin spoon or something that resembles it. Another is returning to a place associated with their addiction. Another common trigger is association with persons with whom the addiction took place. Any of these or other associations can cause strong craving for the drug and severely test the person's resolve to remain abstinent.

One of the most common triggers for relapse is stress. It might be caused by financial problems, marital troubles, the threat of incarceration, difficulties with an employer, or any of the "slings and arrows of outrageous fortune" to which we are all subject. And there is, as almost always, an underlying neurobiologic reason for it; it involves endorphins.

In addition to their vital roles in the experiences of pain and pleasure, there is an additional function that endorphins play. They help us withstand stress. When confronted with danger, we have to quickly decide between "fight or flight." A complex array of chemical changes prepares us for both. The adrenal glands provide both adrenaline and adrenal steroids, to produce the "amped up" effect. To provide a balance, endorphins are released to prevent loss of control. In other words, endorphins act as "mood stabilizers". Once again, an example of exquisite balance.

The problem for those addicted to opiates is that their endorphin systems have been disabled by their addiction. Consider this analogy. To protect a large building from fire, a system is designed to release fire retardant from sprinklers in response to an increase in temperature. An external force, say sunspots, causes the temperature to rise to unprecedented levels, releasing a huge flood of retardant, which causes a lot of damage.

When the force is spent and the clean-up is finished, the decision is made to decrease the sensitivity of the sensors. The force continues intermittently to cause the release of retardant, and the sensitivity of the sensors continues to be decreased. Finally a point is reached where, when a real fire occurs, the sensors and the system are no longer able to respond, and outside sources of the retardant must be purchased and employed.

As a part of the neuroadaptation to the constant injection of large doses of opiates, the brain renders the opiate receptors less responsive to the continuing external heat of heroin doses, making them insensitive to the relatively small amounts of endorphins released by the brain. The addicted brain realizes the imbalance and the lack of response and interprets this as a deficiency of opiates which causes craving. So unless and until the endorphin-receptor system has been completely rehabilitated by prolonged abstinence, the system won't be effective in producing the proper response in a time of stress. The constant heat of addiction has damaged the system, which is the protection against the onset of stress.

So how long does it take to rehabilitate the endorphin system, and how can we tell when it is fully recovered? The answer to both questions is that we just don't know. It is important to keep in mind that because methadone is continuing to interact with the opiate receptors throughout treatment, the endorphin system cannot be rehabilitated while on therapeutic doses of methadone. In order to discontinue methadone treatment, the patient must have the methadone dose slowly decreased so that the brain can recalibrate to each new level. If the taper were proceed too swiftly, the patient will begin to have withdrawal symptoms. Each patient is different, and the pace must be adjusted to the individual's tolerance.

Conclusion

It should be noted that for most of the long history of man's cohabitation with the juice of the poppy on this planet, most societies were able to integrate the use of the material into their culture without significant disruption. China in the nineteenth century is an exception. In contrast, our current struggles to deal with the societal impact of individuals using opiates and other illicit substances, including steroids, demonstrates that in a fundamental way, we have not been able to figure it out. But, for the sake of this presentation, we will leave that to the philosophers and politicians.

The focal point of methadone treatment is not society at large, but rather the individual who has made the decision to try and free him (her) self from the prison of opiate addiction--that same person who made a very bad decision at some point in his life, and followed it up with a long series of bad decisions that led him down the pathway to self-destruction. But, it's not only self-destruction. Heroin and other such addictions destroy relationships, and families, including innocent children. The decision to commit to the long, arduous path to recovery is the beginning of the way back.

There are many responsible ways to seek recovery, and methadone is only one of them. For many reasons it doesn't work for all who try it. The programs are rigid and demanding and the stigma of methadone treatment is a heavy burden to live with. But for some, it is the door they can pass through on the way to reconstructing their lives and embracing the relationships and responsibilities which lead to the gratification that makes our time on this planet worthwhile. The counseling and support provided by well-run programs is critical in helping people learn how to live in the straight world they have been at odds with for so long.

There are at least two things that need improvement. One is access to treatment for everyone who seeks it. The second is wider understanding and compassion for those who still suffer from this affliction. Hopefully, this discussion will be a part of that process.

Methadone has now been successfully used in opiate treatment programs for forty years. The strategy and the patients who have been successful in it have earned more respect than they currently receive.

References

Dole, Vincent, P. Implications of Methadone Maintenance for theories of Narcotic Addiction; JAMA 1988, 260:3025-3029

Nestler, E.M., Aghajanian, G.K. Molecular and Cellular Basis of Addiction; Science, 1997; 278:58-63

Kreek, M.J., Koob, G.F. Drug dependence; stress and dysregulation of brain reward pathways; Drug and Alcohol Dependence 1998; 23-47 National Institutes of Health--Consensus Development Conference Statement; Effective Medical Treatment of Opiate Addiction; 1997

Institute of Medicine; Federal Regulation of Methadone treatment; National Academy Press, Washington 1995.

Nesse, R.M., Berridge, K.C,; Psychoactive Drug Use in Evolutionary Perspective; Science 1997; 27863-66

Messing M.; *The Fix* , University of California Press, 1998

Goldstein, A.; *Addiction; From Biology to Drug Policy;* W.H. Freeman and Co. New York, 1994

Koob, G.F., Lemoal, M.   Drug Abuse: hedonic homeostatic dysregulation. Science 278; 52-58

Chapter 2

The Science and Rationale for Opiate Agonist Treatment

Suma Singh, M.D.

Introduction

Methadone Maintenance is a treatment regimen for the disease of opiate addiction. Patients receive daily doses of methadone (prescription opiate medication) to restore normalcy to a state of relative deficiency of brain opiates. In concept, it is very similar to insulin treatment for diabetes, where patients receive daily doses of insulin (prescription hormone medication) to restore normalcy to a relative deficiency of pancreatic hormone. In this section, the science and clinical rationale for treating opiate addiction with an opiate will be reviewed.

Opiate addiction is a symptom complex (i.e. disease) with physical, emotional, and behavioral consequences resulting from relative deficiency of the naturally occurring opiates (endorphins) in the brain. When viewed in that context, it is not unlike insulin-dependant diabetes – a symptom complex (i.e. disease) of physical, emotional, and behavioral consequences resulting from relative deficiency of a naturally occurring hormone (insulin) in our bodies. Insulin-dependant diabetes can be effectively managed by balancing the body's insulin deficiency with daily injections of a prescription insulin medication, and thereby preventing a host of secondary medical problems associated with poorly controlled diabetes Similarly, opiate dependences (i.e. addiction) can be effectively managed with daily methadone treatment to balance the brain's relative opiate deficiency, allowing patients to function normally and preventing a host of secondary medical problems associated with poorly controlled addiction.

As mentioned previously in this book, the days where drug addiction was perceived as essentially a moral problem or character flaw are behind us. Cumulative scientific evidence gathered over the three past decades clearly establishes that drug addiction is a disease with a physical basis. The data demonstrates that addiction is a disorder of the human brain that severely compromises a patient's ability to regulate and control his/her behaviors (compulsive drug seeking). It has a biological basis in brain just like Parkinson's Disease (dysfunction of the brain's motor system) or Alzheimer's (dysfunction of the brain's cognitive system) or Major Depression (disruption of the brain's mood modulating system). For addiction, the location of the dysfunction has been determined to be in the part of the brain largely responsible for reinforcement and motivation behind basic drives such as hunger, thirst, survival, and well-being.

Dr. Alan Leshner, former Director of the National Institute of Drug Abuse, describes addiction as the drug seizing control of the addicted person's brain, thereby usurping first the mind and then the life...by disrupting receptors and neurotransmitter systems in regions of the brain that normally allow the exercise of choice...resulting in uncontrollable, compulsive drug-seeking and use – the essence of addiction. For the patient with addiction, drug-seeking becomes as primal and instinctual as the need for food and water, often even superceding these basic survival drives. Exercise of intrinsic free choice in the matter becomes nearly impossible at this stage, and external stabilizing intervention becomes necessary.

When Drs. Vincent Dole and Mary Jane Kreek first pioneered the use of methadone to treat opiate addiction in 1963, they postulated the existence of underlying physiological disorder (" a persistent derangement of the endogenous ligand-narcotic receptor system", JAMA 1988) that was treated by methadone and that this was a matter greater than simple substitution or replacement for illicit opioids. Since that time, a great deal of scientific data has illuminated the neurobiological basis for opiate addiction.

Recent data of particular interest are the results of PET scan brain studies of humans with opiate addiction.   Drs. Galynkar and Watras-Ganz completed a preliminary PET scan study (2000) to determine if there were persistent differences in brain function in individuals with opiate addiction compared to individuals who do not have substance abuse, and whether methadone maintenance treatment reduced or reversed these functional abnormalities in the addicted individuals. PET (positron emission tomography) scanning is an imaging tool that evaluates brain function in different regions by measuring the glucose metabolic rate in those regions.   The results revealed a statistically significant difference in glucose metabolic rate in the brains of individuals with opiate addiction compared to individuals without substance use problems.   Additionally, the brain glucose metabolic rate for opiate addicts who had undergone methadone maintenance was intermediate between that of untreated opiate addicts, and individuals without substance use problems.

Based on this data, the authors concluded that neurobiological abnormalities (aberrations in brain function) must exist in the brain of the opiate addict, which persist for several years even after methadone treatment has concluded.   Further research is needed to elucidate the relationship between glucose metabolism rate in the brain, opiate use, and the neuro-chemical abnormalities involved in addictive behavior.

These persistent changes were supported by another PET scan brain study conducted by Drs. Daglish, Weinstein and colleagues from the University of Bristol, United Kingdom.   They used PET scans to measure brain activity by evaluating blood flow in various brain regions. Opiate addicts in stable recovery (abstinence) were placed under the PET scanner and given 2 audiotapes to listen to: one was an autobiographical recording about drug craving (drug stimulus), and the other was a neutral dialogue (neutral stimulus or control group). Results showed that the drug-related stimulus activated 2 specific regions of the brain (left medial prefrontal cortex, left anterior cingulated cortex) and de-activated another region (occipital cortex) when compared to the neutral stimulus. They concluded that these patterns of specific brain-region activation and de-activation reflect the different brain regions influenced by addiction. This study also indicates that these addiction-related brain changes persist even after recovery (stable abstinence from drugs).

In addition to evidence indicating that addiction is associated with fundamental changes in brain's endogenous opiate system and its function, there are also many studies suggesting that the addict's ability to cope with stress is also fundamentally altered. For example, heroin addicts often do not respond, or respond at abnormally low levels to stressful events when actively engaged in their addiction. Addicts that are abstinent and medication-free show exaggerated responses, or excessive susceptibility to stress. In contrast, addicts who are treated with long-term methadone maintenance tend to show a normalization of the stress response, as measured by the body's release of stress hormones. Again, the weight of recent scientific evidence continues to support Dr. Dole's initial theory, that opiate addiction is a persistent derangement of the endogenous ligand-narcotic receptor system, and that opiate agonist treatment is a matter greater than simple substitution or replacement for illicit opioids. Opiate agonist treatment (methadone) appears to normalize the brain's relative opiate deficiency allowing the patient to function more normally.

Since 1963, when Dr. Dole initially hypothesized that heroin addiction was a brain disease with behavioral manifestations, and not just a personality disorder or criminal behavior, 40 years of clinical studies have clearly demonstrated the safety, efficacy, long-term clinical utility of methadone maintenance for opiate addiction. In 1998, the National Institute of Health published a consensus report unequivocally supporting methadone treatment for opiate addiction, and called for measures to increase patient access to this efficacious treatment modality.   The expert panel reviewed an extensive bibliography of 941 references from the National Library of Medicine, MEDLINE and other online databases.

Their conclusions based on overwhelming data supporting reduction in mortality, morbidity, criminality, improved productivity through improved functionality, and public health benefit through reducing HIV/ Hepatitis C viral transmission from injection drug use are as follows:

1. Opiate dependence is a brain-related medical disorder that can be effectively treated with significant benefits for the patient and society, and society must make a commitment to offer effective treatment for opiate dependence to all who need it.
2. All persons dependent on opiates should have access to methadone hydrochloride maintenance therapy under legal supervision, and the US Office of National Drug Control Policy and the US Department of Justice should take the necessary steps to implement this recommendation.
3. There is a need for improved training for physicians and other health care professionals. Training to determine diagnosis and treatment of opiate dependence should also be improved in medical schools.
4. The unnecessary regulations of methadone maintenance therapy and other long-acting opiate agonist treatment programs should be reduced, and coverage for these programs should be a required benefit in public and private insurance programs.

During 2005, internal outcomes data from Santa Clara County Department of Alcohol and Drug Services (DADS) clinics showed more than 75% of patients were effectively treated with low to moderate dose ranges of methadone. Approximately 23% of patients required doses in the higher ranges to achieve stabilization. Of 455 patients enrolled in Methadone Maintenance in DADS clinics during July 2005, more than one half (53%) had demonstrated continuous abstinence from all illicit drugs, active engagement in counseling, absence of criminality, absence of serious behavioral problems, and return to functionality (job, school, etc) for a duration of 1 year or longer. Even more impressively, 34% of DADS methadone maintenance patients had demonstrated all of the above for two consecutive years or longer. Certainly, our own local experience with opiate agonist treatment (methadone maintenance) is congruent with the substantial evidence collected across many US academic and community centers over the past 40 years with respect to the excellent safety, efficacy, clinical utility, and public health benefit attained with this modality.

All patients who suffer from chronic illnesses deserve to be viewed with compassion by both the public and by health professionals. In Dr. Leshner's words, society views with compassion those patients for whom the brain disease is primarily manifested as physical symptoms, such as Parkinson's or Multiple Sclerosis. Society has even learned to accept as legitimate disease, those conditions where brain disease is primarily manifested by emotional symptoms, such as Depression or Schizophrenia. However, those patients with brain diseases where the symptoms are primarily behavioral, such as addiction, are less fortunate.

As addictionologists working with such patients, it is our hope that as science continues to elucidate the relationship between the brain, mind, and behavior, that negative stereotypes and societal stigma showered upon such patients with addiction will be dispelled, so as to improve access for safe and effective treatments to patients who suffer from this disease.

References

Daglish MR, Weinstein A, Malizia AL, Wilson S, Melichar JK, Britten S, Brewer C,

Lingford-Hughs A, Myles JS, Grasby P, Nutt DJ. Changes in regional cerebral blood flow elicited by craving memories in abstinent opiate-dependent subjects.

Kreek MJ   Rationale for maintenance pharmacotherapy in opiate dependence. Res Publ Assoc Res Nerv Ment Dis. 1992. Vol 70. pp 205-230.

Kreek MJ   Methadone-related opiate agonist pharmacotherapy for opiate dependence: Recent molecular and neurochemical research, and future in mainstream medicine. Annals New York Academy of Sciences. 2000. 909: 186-216

NIH Consensus Panel.   Effective medical treatment of opiate addiction. National Consensus Development Panel on Effective Medical Treatment of Opiate Addiction.   JAMA 1998.   Dec 9;280(22):1936-43.

Stimmel B, Kreek MJ   Neurobiology of addictive behaviors and its relationship to methadone maintenance. Mt Sinai Journal of Medicine 2000. Oct-Nov; 67 (5-6): 375-80

Chapter 3

The Behavioral Pharmacology of Methadone:
The Easy-to-Understand Version

Mark Stanford, Ph.D.

Introduction

We'd wake up, find it, no matter how long it takes to find it, and you take it. It's just, one bag weren't enough coz we were sharing it. Then the next bag weren't enough... then we found out it was cheaper to buy a big amount, a bigger amount like a gram... as soon as we found that out then we would smoke as much as we could... It got to the stage where we were just smoking ourselves silly, smoking ourselves to death and it was killing us..." My habit got so high that we... had to sell things... we weren't paying no bills..."

Particularly over the last decade, dramatic advances in the neurosciences have enhanced the understanding of drug addiction. As a result, more people are beginning to understand the nature of addiction and are accepting it as a chronic, relapsing condition that alters normal brain function, just as many other neurological or psychiatric illnesses do.

Research has revealed some major differences between the brains of addicted and nonaddicted individuals and to indicate some common elements of addiction, regardless of the substance used. Science has also provided compelling evidence that the development and manifestation of addiction is influenced by genetic, biological, psychosocial and environmental factors. And, the behaviors of drug addiction are often characterized by an impaired control over drug craving and compulsive continued drug use despite harmful consequences.

Most addictive drugs create the sensations they do because they imitate the brain's natural chemicals, called *neurotransmitters*. Brain cells transmit messages throughout the nervous system when they receive enough of a given neurotransmitter. Addiction to opioid drugs is particularly challenging because the brain produces natural opioid substances and does not discriminate between them and opioid drugs taken externally. The brain's own natural opioids are extremely important for survival and are involved in a variety of behaviors including analgesia, mood, digestion, blood pressure, body temperature, respiration and sleep. They also seem to play an important role within the brain's pleasure/reward system. Interestingly, the brain responds to external opioid drugs, including heroin, as if they are also biologically essential for survival.

When the addiction is established, the brain's own chemistry becomes imbalanced and the nervous system begins to rely on the external opioid to try and regain balance. The problem is, when the external opioid drug is removed by metabolism, the nervous system is left in an unbalanced state resulting in withdrawal pain and craving for more of the drug. The addicted person in this state becomes physically, emotionally and mentally dysfunctional unless and until more opioid drug is taken.

The original methadone research suspected that in many cases, the person addicted to heroin has some kind of physiologic disorder, possibly with an underlying genetic predisposition that manifested itself as compulsive drug seeking/using behaviors after an initial exposure to certain types of drugs. Research then speculated that heroin-induced changes in specific neurobiological systems would persist over long periods and possibly become permanent for some addicts.

At about the same time, observations about the treatment of opioid addiction at the U.S. Public Health Service Hospital in Lexington, Kentucky showed that less than 10% of "hard-core" addicts were able to remain abstinent after treatment from those programs that only offered counseling and psychiatric care. It is now recognized that relapse is one of the hallmarks of addictive disease. Therefore, the newly developing addiction medicine was targeting in on an optimal pharmacological treatment that would complement the psychological and behavioral conditions of opioid addiction.

Since then, some 40 years later, hundreds of research studies from around the world have all confirmed that methadone is soundly based in biologic science and its benefits have been proven in more clinical trials than many drugs used in today's modern medicine. It has helped hundreds of thousands of heroin addicts all over the world. It is both safe and effective for the treatment of opiate addiction.

Even though methadone can be used as an addiction treatment for any of the opioid drugs, its use was initially developed as a pharmacotherapy agent targeting heroin addiction. As such, a review of the basic behavioral pharmacology of heroin will help in the explanation of why methadone is so effective as an addiction medicine.

HEROIN

Heroin addiction: It's like I've got a shotgun in my mouth, my finger's on the trigger and I like the taste of gun metal.

Robert Downey, Jr., Actor

Opioid addicts say that ingesting opiate drugs like heroin calms their nerves, satisfies their cravings and helps them relax. Scientists believe they now know why that might be – ingesting opiate drugs produces major changes in the flow of "feel good" chemicals in the brain, both temporarily and long-term. Heroin is a semisynthetic opiate derived from dried sap of the opium poppy. Also derived from poppy, though not synthesized, are morphine and codeine.

Heroin can be injected, smoked, swallowed or snorted. Intravenous injection produces the greatest intensity and most rapid onset o euphoria. Effects are felt within seconds. Even though effects fo sniffing or smoking develop more slowly, beginning in 10 to 1! minutes, sniffing or smoking heroin has increased in popularity because of the availability of high-purity heroin and the fear of sharing needles. Also, users tend to mistakenly believe that taking heroin ii ways other than IV use will not lead to addiction.

After ingestion, heroin rapidly crosses the blood-brain barrier. The blood-brain barrier is basically a layer of tightly packed cells tha make up the walls of brain capillaries and prevent substances (i.e toxins) in the blood from entering into the brain. These cells selectively filter out the molecules that are allowed to enter the brain creating a more stable, nearly toxin-free environment. However, al psychoactive drugs freely pass the blood brain barrier and enter the brain.

While in the brain, heroin is converted to morphine, which rapidly binds to opioid receptors. Users tend to report feeling a "rush" or a surge of pleasurable sensations. The feeling varies in intensity depending on how much of the drug was ingested and how rapidly the drug enters the brain and binds to the natural opioid receptors. The rush is usually accompanied by a warm flushing of the skin, dry mouth, and a heavy feeling in the user's arms and legs. Following the initial effects, the user will be drowsy for several hours with clouded mental functioning and slow cardiac function. Breathing is slowed, and can possibly slow to the point of death.

Repeated use of heroin produces physical dependency, which means the development of tolerance to the drug's effects that necessitates ever larger amounts of the drug to achieve the same effect. A characteristic withdrawal syndrome upon abrupt cessation of use also develops. Withdrawal symptoms can begin within a few hours of last use and can include restlessness, body ache, muscle pain, insomnia, diarrhea, nausea, stomach cramps, vomiting, and hot/cold flashes. These symptoms peak between 24 and 48 hours after the last dose and subside after about a week, but may persist for up to a month. Heroin withdrawal is generally not fatal in an otherwise healthy adult, but can cause death to the fetus of a pregnant addict.

When purchased on the street, heroin is often adulterated with substances such as sugar, starch, powdered milk, strychnine and other poisons, or other drugs. These additives may not dissolve when injected in a user's system and can clog the blood vessels that lead to the lungs, liver, kidneys, or brain, infecting or even killing patches of cells in vital organs. In addition, many users do not know the heroin's actual strength or its true contents and are at risk of exposure to a tainted or contaminated quantity of heroin causing neurotoxic damage, drug overdose or even death.

Chronic heroin use can lead to medical consequences such as scarred and/or collapsed veins, bacterial infections of the blood vessels and heart valves, abscesses and other soft-tissue infections, and liver or kidney disease. Poor health conditions and depressed respiration from heroin use can cause lung complications, including various types of pneumonia and tuberculosis. Other long-term effects of heroin use can include arthritis and other rheumatologic problems and infection of bloodborne pathogens such as HIV/AIDS and hepatitis B and C (which are contracted by sharing and reusing syringes and other injection paraphernalia). It is estimated that injection drug use has been a factor in one third of all HIV and more than half of all hepatitis C cases in the United States. Heroin use by a pregnant woman can result in a miscarriage or premature delivery. Heroin exposure *in utero* can increase a newborns' risk of SIDS (sudden infant death syndrome).

Opioid Drugs

The term "opioids" includes all of the drugs that come from the opium poppy such as morphine and codeine; semi-synthetics such as heroin; and synthetics such as methadone. The term "opioids" is used to classify a family of substances whose biological action is similar to morphine. These drugs produce a wide range of biological actions including euphoria, pain suppression and sedation, which make them important as medicines. The word *endorphin* is actually the combined form of two words – endogenous (from within) and morphine. The *morphine from within* – endorphin. The pharmacologic action of morphine mimics that of endorphins. There are probably about two dozen different endogenous opioid types that can be categorized in one of three different systems: 1) the **endorphin** system, 2) the **enkephalin** system, and 3) the **dynorphin** system.

Opioid Receptors

Cells found in the nervous system are called *neurons.* Neurons are specialized cells whose main function is to coordinate a wide variety of behaviors using specialized chemical messengers (neurotransmitters) to communicate with other neurons. Neurotransmitters are chemicals that transmit neurological information from neuron to neuron. The neurological information could be about mood, heart rate, blood pressure, movement, remembering something, pleasure, etc. Between each of the brain's 100 billion neurons is a fluid filled space, called a *synapse*, where neurotransmitter messages are sent by neurons and received by other neurons in order to coordinate behavior (figure 1.).

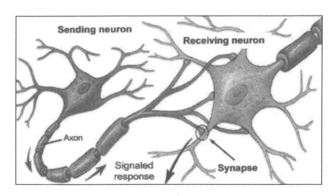

figure 1

Essentially, behavior occurs as a result of neurons releasing neurotransmitters to activate or signal other neurons. Neurons receive this chemical data at their *receptor sites*. If enough receptor sites are stimulated by the chemical data, behavior occurs.

To help understand the biology of behavior including opioid addiction, the "lock and key" model can sometimes assist in describing how neurotransmitters and receptors work. In this model, the neurotransmitter acts like a chemical "key" that fits into and binds to a receptor site "lock". If the correct neurotransmitter *keys* fit into and *unlock* the receptor site, communication between neurons takes place and a behavioral effect results. Exactly what type of behavior is determined by where in the brain this activity occurs and with what type of neurotransmitters, and at which receptor sites. The discovery of specific neurotransmitters and receptors in the brain and body for opiate drugs was central to the discovery of opioid neurotransmitters and then, to the discovery of specific opioid receptor sites. Endorphins are the chemical "keys" for the opiate receptor sites. Endorphins and any type of opiate drug will bind at opiate receptors and signal a response. Receptors are located along the outer membrane of the neuron. (figure 2)

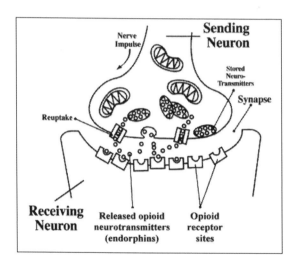

figure 2

Three of the most studied opioid receptor sites are the *mu, delta* and *kappa* receptors, named using the letters of the Greek alphabet to differentiate each type. The *mu* opioid receptor site has received the most attention because it tells us a lot about how opioid drugs work.

Some drugs bind with greater strength (affinity) at receptor sites than others and will produce a more pronounced effect. For example heroin has a greater affinity for binding at the *mu, delta and kappa* opiate receptor sites than morphine. These opioid receptors are associated with mood and pleasure, among other things. Because heroin binds more readily at these sites, it produces a more intense behavioral euphoric effect.

Methadone Treatment

Because heroin isn't just a drug to users, it's an abiding personal passion and an all consuming concern, a soothing balm of oblivion to calm the dull ache of existence. It's the reason some people get up in the morning and the reason they fall asleep at night. It's the first thought they think of when they realize they're awake, alive, or alone. It's an identity, vocation, and pastime, a lover, master, and friend. In fact, heroin is just about everything to every addict, all the time. Everything, that is, except safe, legal, and free.

Anonymous

Research from the National Institute of Drug Abuse (NIDA) has shown that opioid dependent individuals will compulsively continue to use opioids despite adverse physical, emotional and life altering consequences because of at least two motivational factors: 1) the desire to self medicate the pain of narcotic withdrawal symptoms, and 2) the driving force of drug craving.

The primary goal of methadone treatment is to stabilize clients on a sufficient dose of methadone to both treat the symptoms of withdrawal and to block the behaviors of drug craving – two precipitating dynamics for relapse behaviors. Once stabilized, clients can then begin the process of recovery by gaining new skills from counseling that will enable them to regain a normal lifestyle. As used in maintenance treatment, methadone is not a heroin substitute. It is important to understand that methadone does not actually "replace" or "substitute" for other opioids. That's why the terms replacement and/or substitution therapy are inaccurate and misleading. Instead, these medications are able to suspend withdrawal symptoms, decrease drug craving behaviors and block the actions from other opioid drugs such as heroin.

The pharmacological effects of methadone are markedly different from those of heroin. Injected, snorted, or smoked, heroin causes an almost immediate "rush" or brief period of euphoria that wears off quickly, terminating in a "crash." The cycle of euphoria, crash, and craving repeated several times a day leads to a cycle of addiction and severe behavioral disruption.

These characteristics of heroin use result from the drug's rapid onset of action and its short duration of action in the brain. An individual who uses heroin multiple times per day subjects the brain and body to marked, rapid fluctuations as the opiate effects come and go (figure 3).

The individual also will experience an intense craving for more heroin to stop the cycle, fend off withdrawal and to reinstate the euphoria. Ultimately however, when tolerance to the drug has been established, the addicted person continues to use to avoid the pain of drug withdrawal and to feel relatively normal.

Methadone has a very gradual and slow onset of action compared with heroin. Because of this, patients stabilized on methadone do not experience the euphoric "rush" (figure 4).

Methadone is metabolized more slowly than heroin and thereby allows the brain and body to avoid the stressful ups and downs caused by heroin. When on a stabilized dose during maintenance treatment, there is also a marked reduction of the desire and craving for heroin.

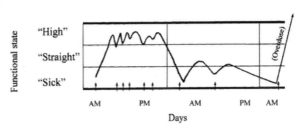

figure 3

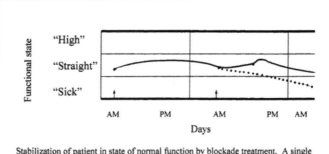

figure 4

Essentially all physiological systems are affected by opiate addiction. A characteristic syndrome occurs when an opiate addict goes through withdrawal. This syndrome includes perspiration, tremor, gooseflesh, restlessness, myalgia, anorexia, nausea, vomiting, abdominal cramps, diarrhea, fever, hyperpnea, and hypertension. Persistent symptoms such as sleep disturbances, irritability, restlessness, and poor concentration can continue for months or longer after the drug use has stopped.

On one level, opioid dependency is an adaptation of the body to opiates. With repeated use, dependence develops when the body's various systems have adapted to the opioid where they require the drug to regulate a physiological balance.

Methadone, as used in the treatment of opioid addiction, has an affinity for *mu* opioid receptors in the brain where it blocks the withdrawal syndrome and diminishes craving behaviors which otherwise can lead to continued illicit drug use.

Of importance is the fact that at *mu* receptor sites, methadone will also block the effects of other opioid drugs including heroin. This means that even if a patient on methadone ingests heroin, the blocking effect will disallow any heroin action and the patient is prevented from what might have otherwise been a long and torturous relapse.

An Optimal Dose For Methadone Maintenance

There have been many research studies comparing various doses of methadone for maintenance treatment. Reports have consistently shown that patients receiving higher doses of methadone compared to those receiving lower doses have much better outcomes – where outcomes are defined in terms of abstinence from illicit opioid use, length of treatment stay, and overall improvement in the quality of life.

Essentially, all of the research on dosing has concluded that there is no evidence of lower doses being adequate for the vast majority of patients. Vincent Dole, one of the co-discoverers of methadone for the treatment of opioid addiction, stated, "There is no compelling reason for prescribing doses that are only marginally adequate. As with antibiotics, the prudent policy is to give enough medication to ensure success".
(see figure 5).

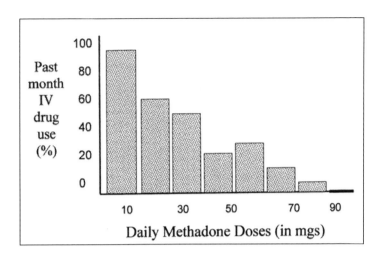

Figure 5

More recently, Payte (2002) noted, "Arbitrary dose ceilings have no foundation in science or clinical medicine. Programs with 'dose caps' can expect problems with accreditation." Furthermore, the U.S. federal regulations or addiction medicine associations do not endorse such "caps".

In terms of safety, a meta-analysis of methadone dosing studies found that patients having access to "high-dose maintenance" were actually at a greater reduced risk of fatal heroin overdose during treatment compared with those at lower doses. Remember, the goal of methadone is to stabilize the opioid addicted person so that withdrawal pain and drug craving behaviors are suspended. The optimal dose amount to initiate and maintain stabilization depends on individual patient needs.

A Chronic, Relapsing Disorder

According to Alan Leshner, past President for the National Institute of Drug Abuse, "Addiction is rarely an acute illness. For most people, it is a chronic, relapsing disorder. Total abstinence for the rest of one's life is a relatively rare outcome from a single treatment episode.

Relapses are more the norm. Thus, addiction must be approached more like other chronic illnesses—such as diabetes and chronic hypertension—than like an acute illness, such as bacterial infection of a broken bone. This requirement has tremendous implications for how we understand and ultimately evaluate treatment effectiveness and treatment outcomes. Viewing addiction as a chronic, relapsing disorder means that a good treatment outcome, and the most reasonable expectation, is a significant decrease in drug use and long periods of abstinence, with only occasional relapses. That makes a reasonable standard for treatment success—as is the case for other chronic illness—the management of the illness, not a cure".

Since 1965, methadone maintenance programs have proved to be the most effective treatment for opiate (e.g., heroin) addiction. Under medical supervision, a daily dose of 60-100 mg of methadone prevents withdrawal symptoms and drug craving behaviors, produces no euphoria, and allows patients the opportunity to return to a lifestyle free of the need for compulsive drug seeking and use.

The effectiveness of methadone treatment has also been demonstrated extensively by remarkable reductions in criminal arrests, increases in employment, and stability of social relationships.

References

Ball, J.C. and Ross, A. (1994). The Effectiveness of Methadone Maintenance Treatment. New York: Springer-Verlag.

Borg L, Kreek MJ. The pharmacology of opioids. In: Graham AW, Schultz TK, Mayo-Smith MF, Ries

Caplehorn, J.R.M. (1994). A comparison of abstinence-oriented and indefinite methadone maintenance treatment. International Journal of the Addictions 29(11): 1361-1375.

Dole VP, Nyswander ME, Kreek MJ. Narcotic blockade. Arch Int Med. 1966;118:304-309.

Goldstein, A.; Tachibana, S.; Lowney, L.I.; Hunkapiller M. and Hood, L. Dynorphin-(1-13), an extraordinary potent opioid peptide. Proceedings of the National Academy of Science USA 1979 76: 6666-6670.

Hughes, J. Isolation of an endogenous compound from the brain with properties similar to morphine. Brain Research 1975 (a), 88: 295-308

Kosten TR, George TP. The neurobiology of opioid dependence: implications for treatment. Science & Practice Perspectives. 2002;1(1):13-20.

Leshner, A.I. *Addiction is a brain disease, and it matters.* Science *278:45-47. 1997.*

Nestler, EJ, Malenka RC. The addicted brain. Scientific American. March 2004.

NIH (National Institutes of Health). Effective Medical Treatment of Opiate Addiction. NIH Consensus Statement. Bethesda, MD: National Institutes of Health; 1997 (Nov 17-19);15(6):1-38. (See also: JAMA. 1998;280:1936-1943.)

Payte JT, Zweben JE, Martin J. Opioid maintenance treatment. In: Graham AW, Schultz TK, Mayo-Smith MF, Ries RK, Wilford BB. Principles of Addiction Medicine. Chevy Chase, MD: American Society of Addiction Medicine; 2003: 751-766.

Woods, J. How methadone works. National Alliance of Methadone Advocates. 2003

Chapter 4

Effectiveness of Methadone Treatment: A Review of Outcomes

Joan E. Zweben, Ph.D.

Over 40 years of research documents the efficacy of methadone, particularly its impact on issues of public health and safety. Methadone treatment has been shown to reduce illicit drug use and drug-associated crime; slow the spread of HIV and facilitate intervention for hepatitis C (HCV); and improve health status, neonatal outcomes, psychiatric status, participation in employment, and family functioning. As emphasis grows on the importance of using treatments based on research evidence, the extensive literature on a variety of outcomes has helped reduce the stigma and other barriers to access.

In order to understand the effects of treatment, it is important to have a picture of the natural history of a disorder if it is untreated or inadequately treated. Thus one of the most important studies is not about methadone treatment at all (Hser, Hoffman, Grella, & Anglin, 2001). It is a longitudinal study of heroin users that examined their drug use, health and mental health issues, employment patterns, criminal behavior and mortality. The study focused on 581 male heroin users who were admitted to the California Civil Addict

Program between 1962-1964, and have been followed since that time by UCLA researchers. Follow-up rates were exceptionally high only 12 were lost to follow up. Very few participants were on methadone, and thus the study shows the natural history of heroin addiction (in males), when methadone treatment is not utilized.

The 33-year follow up (1996-1997) revealed that 49% were dead and most of the rest were doing poorly. Many were using heroin and other drugs, drinking alcohol daily, and smoking tobacco. They had high rates of health problems and criminal justice involvement, and psychological distress. Of those who were alive, only 20%-22% were abstinent, and these participants had less criminal involvement, health problems and better health and employment status.

The outcome data on methadone patients provides a striking contrast Methadone patients have been extensively studied, in part because the legal requirement that they obtain their medication from special clinics means they are a favorite for researchers. It is possible to locate and follow methadone patients more easily than participants in other types of programs. A voluminous research base permits us to examine a variety of questions, and over long periods of time. Many of the early studies were done before it was widely accepted that persons with the history necessary to qualify for methadone treatment are unlikely to be able to discontinue and preserve their gains. Thus it is possible to examine the trajectories for patients who remain in treatment, who discontinue voluntarily, and who are involuntarily tapered from the medication. Those who remain on medication continue to improve and maintain their gains, with some continuing to improve over a period of years. While those who discontinue voluntarily do somewhat better than those who do not, by the end of a year, they too have relapsed.

This is consistent with the expectations of Drs. Dole and Nyswander, who state that methadone is necessary to correct brain chemistry anomalies. It normalizes but does not cure a dysfunction, in much the same way that thyroid medication restores thyroid function. Methadone is a relatively inexpensive medication. Much of the costs are associated with compliance with a complex set of regulations. It is ikely that the costs of indefinite maintenance on methadone will be significantly reduced as research continues to clarify the pace at which psychosocial services can be reduced, and as regulations are simplified. Current models support the view that well-functioning patients can be transitioned to physicians in office-based practice. This is called "medical maintenance" and is supported by 20 years' research evidence. Federal and state regulatory barriers currently prevent full implementation of these findings, but efforts are underway to update regulations in the light of scientific findings.

Reduction of Illict Drug Use and Drug-Associated Crime

One of the most striking benefits of methadone treatment is a dramatic reduction in both illicit drug use and drug-associated crime (Ball & Ross, 1991). A variety of studies have documented rapid drops at the outset of methadone treatment, with continuing improvement over a period of several years. Some important "natural experiments" occurred during the 1980's, when methadone treatment was abruptly discontinued in several California counties. Thanks to the adeptness of UCLA researchers, it was shown that the relatively low crime rates of patients in treatment jumped immediately for those unable to find a means of continuing to receive methadone. It remained low for those able to find a way to stay in treatment. Many other studies show a drop in crime within the first few months of entering methadone treatment.

It is important to understand that much benefit is obtained by relieving drug craving, but coping patterns take time to undo. Patients who do not extricate themselves from networks of drug users involved in criminal activity are at higher risk of relapse, and also are more likely to avoid learning prosocial behaviors. For example, lying is a ubiquitous pattern in those who are currently using drugs. It is common for drug use to be discontinued, but lying remains tempting as a way of dealing with conflict with one's partner, friends, or employers. Participation in counseling and self help groups makes it more likely that a commitment to honesty will be seen as part of the recovery process, and that patients will disengage from social networks of users. This is one of a number of reasons that criminal behavior tends to continue to decrease after the initial reductions.

In recent years, the gains possible for methadone patients have been undercut by the spread of cocaine into most urban environments and many rural ones. A criminal history that is not related to drug use and cocaine use are two factors that reduce treatment effectiveness among methadone patients. Cocaine use has remained a challenging problem for most programs.

Improvement in Health Status

Methadone patients have a 4-8 fold reduction in death rate compared to those untreated. Reductions in various types of illness also occurs because many of those in treatment are able to extricate themselves from the health hazards of a drug using life style, and access to physicians in the clinics provides some opportunity for early referral for emergent problems. Programs that can offer comprehensive physical and mental health services show significantly better outcomes for their patients. Although it would seem that programs that were part of large-scale medical systems would be better able to provide comprehensive care, barriers within such systems often deter such efforts. Clinics must have the resources to advocate vigorously for good care for their patients, and to closely coordinate that care once it is available.

Ironically, the advent of the HIV epidemic in 1978 made methadone treatment visible in a positive way and resulted in a re-examination of issues previously buried under the stigma. The new emphasis on a public health perspective brought a re-examination of attitudes and practices. Studies of HIV in injection drug users indicate that the longer a group of patients was in MMT, the lower the seropositivity for the HIV virus. Although some patients in MMT do engage in risky behavior and acquire the virus, HIV conversion is lower in MMT patients than those outside methadone treatment. Studies showed that patients who were not in treatment were injecting drugs, sharing needles, visiting shooting galleries and practicing unsafe sex at significantly higher rates than those in treatment. Clinics are currently a major point of intervention to teach risk reduction techniques and expedite referral to treatment for the HIV virus.

The influence of a public health perspective has not only helped to reduce the stigma, it has opened the possibility of new ways of thinking about treatment goals. HIV service providers quickly pointed out that many drug users had little or no commitment to stop their drug use. Extensive studies on interventions to reduce the spread of the HIV virus demonstrated that harm reduction approaches were effective. Methadone treatment providers have always struggled with meeting the needs of patients with very different goals. Some were committed to complete abstinence from illicit drugs and alcohol; others merely wanted to reduce the hassle associated with using. The harm reduction framework allows programs to work with those who are not committed to abstinence within a model that does not define their efforts as failure if the patient does not abstain. This improved the morale of the treatment providers, and allowed them to maintain a positive relationship with their patients. It also produced demonstrable benefits in public health.

The hepatitis C virus (HCV) is more highly transmissible, and many patients are HCV positive upon entry into treatment. Among injection drug users in California, rates run 85%-90%. Recent efforts to treat HCV have been successful in methadone patients, even if they still use some drugs, so long as they are not engaged in daily use (Sylvestre, Litwin, Clements, & Gourevitch, 2005). Many methadone patients are still not aware that treatment can be effective, and avoid getting initial testing or completing an appropriate workup. Peer based education (using videos) and psychoeducational support groups are under investigation as key elements in engaging patients and supporting them through the ordeal of treating their HCV.

It is generally agreed that partly due to the aging of the population in treatment, patients today are far more medically ill and require more resources than before. Cutbacks in resources for medical care have a significant impact on the program's ability to meet the medical needs of its patients.

Improvement in Psychiatric and Psychosocial Functioning

As in other modalities of addiction treatment, co-occurring disorders are the norm, not the exception. In fact there is some evidence that heroin users who seek treatment have higher rates of psychiatric disorders such as depression than those who do not. Mood and anxiety disorders (especially Post Traumatic Stress Disorder, or PTSD) are the most common. Psychotic conditions unrelated to drug use are relatively uncommon, but most clinics have a small number of severely mentally ill patients enrolled in their programs. In general methadone is compatible with psychotropic medications, though some must be carefully monitored. Appropriate treatment of a co-existing psychiatric condition improves treatment outcome. Unfortunately many clinics to not have the resources to address such conditions effectively. It is increasingly common for counseling staff to be exposed to cognitive behavioral techniques supported by research evidence. It is unclear how well they are prepared to implement these interventions. Although research-based interventions for PTSD exist, they generally require a higher level of clinical skill and it is unusual to find specific program components within clinics, despite the high prevalence of this disorder in both men and women.

Employment, pursuit of education, and family functioning are key psychosocial indicators that improve when given appropriate forms of attention. Enhanced services result in improvement in these areas, especially if there is a tight fit between the specific services offered and the patient's problem profile (McLellan, Arndt, Metzger, Woody, & O'Brien, 1993; McLellan et al., 1997; McLellan et al., 1998). Although both accreditation and state regulations stress the importance of using a focused treatment plan to guide counseling sessions, counselors report that complex demands for documentation reduce the time they have available to attend to patient needs. Case management becomes increasingly difficult as community resources are lost.

Cost-Benefit Studies

Cost-benefit studies repeatedly show that the benefits of methadone treatment outweigh the costs. The large California CALDATA

Gerstein, Johnson, Harwood, Suter, & Malloy, 1994) study released
n 1994 indicated that methadone treatment showed the greatest
savings of all existing treatment and recovery modalities studied. The
study found a ratio of 1:10, meaning that $10 was saved for every $1
invested in treatment. Other studies, usually focusing on single
episodes of treatment, report similar findings. A recent study that used
a lifetime simulation model found a benefit-cost ratio of 1:38 (Zarkin,
Dunlap, Hicks, & Mamo, 2005). This model factors in existing data
where possible to create a lifetime model more compatible with the
view of addiction as a chronic disorder characterized by relapse over
time, rather than an acute problem that can be addressed in a single
treatment episode.

Key Outside Reviews

There are three outside scientific reviews that played a significant role
in reducing the stigma and encouraging effective treatment. In 1990,
the Government Accounting Office (Government Accounting Office,
1990) (since renamed Government Accountability Office) conducted a
study of methadone programs and produced a striking finding about
dosing. Although the National Institute on Drug Abuse had
documented that 60 mg methadone was a minimum adequate dose, 21
of the 24 programs studied had average doses below that. Often,
physicians were constrained by "program policy" and could not
prescribe appropriate doses. Subsequent research documented that
increasing the dose of methadone resulted in greatly improved
retention and reductions in drug use. Doses of 80 mg and above
produced the best outcomes, with much higher doses required by some
patients. Unfortunately, it is still not unusual to find patients,
clinicians and program administrators attempting to make a virtue out
of low doses. Patients vary enormously in their level of opiate
tolerance and dependence, and in how well they absorb, metabolize
and eliminate the medication. Doses must be individualized and not
limited by "policy." If a patient is continuing to use opiates, the first
question should be whether he or she is taking an adequate dose, as
that will dominate or undermine other factors in producing
improvement.

The second milestone was the publication of an Institute of Medicine (IOM) report on the Federal Regulation of Methadone Treatment (Rettig & Yarmolinsky, 1995). The IOM is chartered by the National Academy of Sciences. This highly prestigious committee concluded that the effectiveness of methadone treatment is well established, but overregulation created barriers to access and implementation of good practices. They examined the impact of diversion, the issue that inspired much of the early regulations. After careful study, they concluded that the risks of diversion and misuse did not warrant the unusual level of regulation, and that these needed to be modified to promote better access and good care.

The third milestone was the convening of an NIH Consensus Development Conference in 1997 (National Consensus Development Panel on Effective Medical Treatment of Opiate Addiction, 1998). This process has been crafted by NIH to address controversial topics in medicine and public health in an unbiased, impartial manner. An independent panel of non-federal professionals in health fields is convened to hear reports by experts, who present research on specific aspects of the topic. After discussion, the panel issues findings and recommendations. The panel reviewed the existing medical literature and attended a series of expert presentations, and then strongly recommended broader access to methadone treatment, through reduction of regulatory barriers and active leadership in addressing stigma and other issues.

Conclusion

In summary, methadone treatment has been exhaustively studied from a variety of perspectives. Although inappropriate policies and practices can undermine its effectiveness, when properly implemented it is a powerful tool to bring improvement in measures of public health and safety.

References

Ball, J., & Ross, A. (1991). *The Effectiveness of Methadone Maintenance Treatment*. New York: Springer-Verlag.

ierstein, D. R., Johnson, R. A., Harwood, H. J., Suter, N., & Malloy, K. (1994). *CALDATA: Evaluating Recovery Services -- The California Drug and Alcohol Treatment Assessment.* Sacramento, Ca.: California Department of Alcohol and Drug Programs.

iovernment Accounting Office. (1990). *Methadone Maintenance* (No. GAO/HRD-90-104 (1990)). Washington D.C.: General Accounting Office.

Iser, Y. I., Hoffman, V., Grella, C. E., & Anglin, M. D. (2001). A 33-year follow-up of narcotics addicts. *Arch Gen Psychiatry, 58*(5), 503-508.

McLellan, A. T., Arndt, I. O., Metzger, D. S., Woody, G. E., & O'Brien, C. P. (1993). The effects of psychosocial services in substance abuse treatment. *Journal of the American Medical Association, 269*(15), 1953-1959.

McLellan, A. T., Grisson, G. R., Zanis, D., Randall, M., Brill, P., & O'Brien, C. P. (1997). Problem-service matching in addiction treatment. *Archives of General Psychiatry, 54*, 730-735.

McLellan, A. T., Hagan, T. A., Levine, M., Gould, F., Meyers, K., Bencivengo, M., et al. (1998). Supplemental social services improve outcomes in public addiction treatment. *Addiction, 93*(10), 1489-1499.

National Consensus Development Panel on Effective Medical Treatment of Opiate Addiction. (1998). Effective medical treatment of opiate addiction. *Journal of the American Medical Association, 280*(22), 1936-1943.

Rettig, R. A., & Yarmolinsky, A. (1995). *Federal Regulation of Methadone Treatment.* Washington D.C.: National Academy Press.

Sylvestre, D. L., Litwin, A. H., Clements, B. J., & Gourevitch, M. N. (2005). The impact of barriers to hepatitis C virus treatment in recovering heroin users maintained on methadone. *Journal of Substance Abuse Treatment, 29*, 159-165.

Zarkin, G. A., Dunlap, L. J., Hicks, K. A., & Mamo, D. (2005). Benefits and costs of methadone treatment: results from a lifetime simulation model. *Health Economics, 14*, 1133-1150.

Chapter 5

Effectiveness of Methadone as a Medical Treatment for Opioid Addiction

Judith Martin, M.D.

Key Questions About Methadone Maintenance Treatment

Medical interventions are judged first by their safety and by their efficacy. Of course, price, and ease of administration also matter. For example, even a very safe and effective medication would not be very popular if it had to be delivered by intravenous infusion, of if it cost a thousand dollars a day. But the most important questions that medical researchers answer when they study a medication are: Does it work? Is it safe?

The questions that patients ask about methadone reflect these concerns: How is methadone better for me than using heroin? What are the side effects? Will it take care of my craving for drugs? Substantial research over 40 years answers these questions. We should make it clear, though, that outcome statistics for methadone maintenance are not just about the medication. There is no such thing as 'just methadone' in the treatment of addiction in the US.

Methadone maintenance in the United States is delivered in specially licensed facilities called Opioid Treatment Programs (OTPs). (Other names for these programs are Narcotic Treatment Programs, or methadone clinics.) Because the OTP is strictly regulated, methadon maintenance is delivered in a particular way that meets Federal an State regulations, and sometimes has nothing to do with evidence based research. There is mandated counseling, and mandated urin testing, as well as daily observation by nurses while the patient take the dose at the window.

What Is A Good Outcome For Opiate Addiction Treatment?

Addiction is a chronic illness, so we don't have a cure for it. Howeve good addiction treatment controls the disease and prevents the long term ravages to the person's life. Control of the addiction include control of the behaviors that are part of the disease, so when we loo at outcomes we use a broad lens.

In addiction treatment, even such non-medical things such as stayin out of jail, becoming employed, and getting along with one's spous are taken into account as positive outcomes of treatment. Of course we also study whether the patient continues to use drugs, or ha reduced or eliminated illicit or harmful use of substances.

Because addiction is chronic, good outcomes come with ongoing care If treatment is interrupted, relapse may occur. So one of the measure of a good outcome is whether the patient has remained in treatment This is called treatment retention.

The following table summarizes some of the outcomes we look for i addiction treatment.

Table 1

Desired outcomes for addiction treatment
Retention in treatment
Reduction or discontinuation of the use of illicit or harmful substances
Reduction in mortality
Increase in productive activities and employment
Improvement in family and social relationships

| prevention of addiction-related diseases such as HIV or abscesses or endocarditis |
| improvement in emotional and psychiatric health |
| improvement in self-efficacy and personal growth (spiritual health) |
| Reduction in criminal activities |

Some of these outcomes are hard to measure, such as personal growth, or family relationships. Some of these outcomes are measured by comparing how the person is doing before treatment to how he or she is doing during treatment. Other outcomes compare persons who are actively using drugs and not in treatment, to those who are now in treatment, as a group.

What Outcomes Have Been Measured For Methadone Maintenance Treatment?

Here are some of the outcomes that have actually been measured for methadone maintenance treatment:

Table 2

Outcomes for Methadone Maintenance Treatment

- 8-10 fold reduction in death rate
- reduction of drug use
- reduction of criminal activity
- engagement in socially productive roles
- reduced spread of HIV
- excellent retention

One way of saying this is: the patient's life becomes stabilized by this treatment. The medication becomes a platform that allows the patient to live his or her life, and engage in recovery activities. A legal, steady, long-acting dose of prescribed daily methadone stabilizes the brain opiate receptors and allows normalization of brain function, so the patient starts 'acting normal.'

Reduction In Medical Problems By Methadone Maintenance Treatment

Some of the benefits of methadone maintenance treatment are related to reduction in illness, whether related to opiates or to other dangerous practices that are tied to active addiction.

For example, stopping injection drug use reduces admissions to hospitals for abscesses or other skin infections, or endocarditis (heart infection). It has been very clearly documented that methadone maintenance treatment reduces the sero-conversion to HIV.
In the case of pregnant women on MMT, babies will be born healthier by avoiding heroin.

As shown above in the outcomes table, MMT saves lives (reduces the death rate, or mortality). Most of these addiction-related deaths are opiate overdoses, when actively addicted persons inject too much heroin at one time and stop breathing.

Table 3

Medical problems related to opiate addiction
Opiate overdose and death
HIV infection from contaminated needles. Patients may develop AIDS.
Hepatitis B or C from contaminated needles, cookers, cotton, water. Chronic hepatitis may lead to cirrhosis and liver failure.
Endocarditis (heart infection) from contaminated injection into the bloodstream. Heart valves are destroyed and may require open heart surgery.
Abscess or cellulitis from contaminated needle injection into the skin and subcutaneous tissue. May require incision and drainage, or IV antibiotics.
Necrotizing fasciitis from contaminated needles. Large areas of skin and muscle tissue may be lost, even if the patient survives.
Botulism from contaminated black tar heroin. Botulism toxin causes paralysis, and the patient may stop breathing.

| remature labor and low birth weight from heroin abuse. |
| Daily discomfort from withdrawal symptoms. These include achiness, sweating, diarrhea, nasal congestion, stomach cramps, nausea, irritability, tremors, etc. |
| Insomnia from withdrawal symptoms. |

Every one of the medical problems on this table except one is prevented by methadone maintenance treatment. Hepatitis C is the exception. The reason for this is that most patients already have used needles at least a few times, and already have hepatitis C by the time they come in for treatment. Hepatitis C is very contagious, and it doesn't take long to be exposed. Methadone maintenance treatment would prevent hepatitis C in patients who have not yet used needles, for example young people who 'snort' heroin, or smoke it.

Efficacy References

Appel, P. W., H. Joseph, et al. (2001). "Selected in-treatment outcomes of long-term methadone maintenance treatment patients in New York State." The Mount Sinai Journal of Medicine 68(No. 1): 55-51.

Ball, J. C. and A. Ross (1991). The Effectiveness of Methadone Maintenance Treatment. New York, Springer-Verlag.

Gronbladh, L., L. S. Ohlund, et al. (1990). "Mortality in heroin addiction: impact of methadone treatment." Acta Psychiatr Scand 82(3): 223-7.

Acta Psychiatr Scand, September 1, 1990; 82(3): 223-7.

MEDLINE ABSTRACT

The mortality within a cohort of 115 street heroin addicts was studied for 5-8 years using the Kaplan-Meier survival estimate technique. This differed markedly from the relatively low mortality of 166 comparable heroin addicts given methadone maintenance treatment (MT). The street addicts' mortality rate was 63 times that expected, compared with official statistics for a group of this age and sex distribution. When 53 patients in MT were involuntarily expelled from treatment, due to violation of programme rules, they returned to the high mortality of street addicts (55 times the expected). A group of 34 rehabilitated patients who left MT with medical consent retained the low mortality of MT patients (their mortality rate was times that expected). Despite this great improvement in survival, even patients in MT showed a moderately elevated mortality (8 times the expected), mainly due to diseases acquired before entering the treatment programme. It is concluded that MT exerts a major improvement in the survival of heroin addicts.

Langendam, M., G. vanBrussel, et al. (2001). "The impact of harm reduction-based methadone treatment on mortality among heroin users." Am J Public Health **91**(5): 774-80.

MEDLINE ABSTRACT

OBJECTIVES: The purpose of this study was to investigate the impact of harm-reduction-based methadone programs on mortality among heroin users. METHODS: A prospective cohort investigation was conducted among 827 participants in the Amsterdam Cohort Study. Poisson regression was used to identify methadone maintenance treatment characteristic (dosage, frequency of program attendance, and type of program) that are significantly and independently associated with mortality due to natural causes and overdose. RESULTS: From 1985 to 1996, 89 participants died of natural causes, and 31 died as a result of an overdose. After adjustment for HIV and underweight status, there was an increase in natural-cause mortality among subjects who left methadone treatment (relative risk [RR] = 2.38, 95% confidence interval [CI] = 1.28, 4.55). Leaving treatment was also related to higher overdose mortality, but only among injection drug users (RR = 4.55, 95% CI = 1.89, 10.00). CONCLUSIONS: Harm-reduction-based methadone treatment, in which the use of illicit drugs is tolerated, is strongly related to decreased mortality from natural causes and from overdoses. Provision of methadone in itself, together with social-medical care, appears more important than the actual methadone dosage.

Medical Comorbidity References

Garfein, R., D. Vlahov, et al. (1996). "Viral infections in short- term injection drug users: the prevalence of the hepatitis C, hepatitis B, human immunodeficiency, T-lympho tropic viruses." Am J Public Health **86**: 655-661.

lagan, H. and D. C. D. Jarlais (2000). "HIV and HCV Infection mong Injecting Drug Users." the Mount Sinai journal of medicine 7(Nos. 5&6): 423-428.

Metzger, D. S., G. E. Woody, et al. (1993). "Human Immunodeficiency virus seroconversion among drug users in- and out f-treatment: And 18-month prospective follow-up." Journal of Acquired Immune Deficiency Syndrome 6: 1049-1056.

Noone, M., M. Tabaqchali, et al. (2002). "*Clostridium novyi* causing Necrotizing fasciitis in an injecting drug user." Journal of Clinical Pathology 55: 141-142.

Novick, D. M. (2000). "The impact of hepatitis C virus infection on methadone maintenance treatment." The Mount Sinai Journal of Medicine 67(5 & 6): 437-443.

Novick, D. M., H. Joseph, et al. (1990). "Absence of antibody to human immunodeficiency virus in long-term, socially rehabilitated methadone maintenance patients." Arch Intern Med 150(1): 97-9.

Human immunodeficiency virus (HIV) infection has become widespread among parenteral drug abusers. We measured antibody to HIV and hepatitis B virus markers in 58 long-term, socially rehabilitated methadone-maintained former heroin addicts. None of the 58 had antibody to HIV, but one or more markers of hepatitis B virus infection were seen in 53 (91%). The duration of methadone maintenance was 16.9 +/- 0.5 years, and the median dose of methadone was 60 mg (range, 5 to 100 mg). Before methadone treatment, the patients had abused heroin parenterally for 10.3 +/- 1.7 years, and they had engaged in additional high-risk practices for HIV infection. We conclude that successful outcomes during methadone maintenance treatment are associated with sparing of parenteral drug abusers from HIV infection.

Smolyakov, R., K. Riesenberg, et al. (2002). "Streptococcal Septic Arthritis and Necrotizing Fasciitis in an Intravenous Drug User Couple Sharing Needles." IMAJ 4: 302-303.

Sullivan, L. and D. A. Fiellin (2004). "Hepatitis C and HIV Infections: Implications for Clinical Care in Injection Drug Users." The American Journal on Addictions 13: 1-20.

Our objective is to provide a state-of-the-art review on hepatitis C (HCV) and the human immunodeficiency virus (HIV) in injection drug use (IDUs), highlighting important clinical issues. We performed a literatu review from the MEDLINE database for research from 1966 to 2003, wit an emphasis on recent consensus documents. Of the estimated 15 millio illicit drug users in the U.S., approximately 1.0 to 1.5 million inject drug IDUs are at significant risk of contracting HCV and HIV, with IDL accounting for 60% of new HCV cases and 25% of new HIV infections. is a major risk factor for HCV/HIV coinfection, which significantly impac on each disorder's progression. It appears that treatment response in IDL with HCV or HIV is similar to non-IDUs with these viruses and tha medication adherence and treatment outcomes are optimized when linke with substance abuse treatment. Providers caring for patients who are c were IDUs must be aware of the management of these diseases and mak efforts to integrate their medical care with the treatment of their substanc abuse.

Werner, S. B., D. Passaro, et al. (2000). "Wound Botulism i California, 1951-1998: Recent Epidemic in Heroin Injectors." Clinica Infectious Diseases **31**: 1018-1024

Chapter 6

Co-Occurring Mental Health Issues

Ali Alkoraishi, M.D.

Introduction

A person who has both substance abuse and psychiatric problems is said to have a *dual diagnosis*, sometimes also called, co-occurring disorders. To recover fully, the person needs treatment for both problems.

Prevalence of The Problem

There is a lack of information on the exact numbers of people with a dual diagnosis, but research has shown that it is not that uncommon. According to reports published in the *Journal of the American Medical Association (JAMA)*:

- Of all people diagnosed as mentally ill, 29% currently abuse either alcohol or drugs and 60% will abuse either alcohol or other drugs some time during their lifetime.

- Roughly 50 percent of individuals with severe mental disorders are affected by substance abuse.

- Adults with a substance use disorder in 2002 were almost three times as likely to have serious mental illness (20. percent) as those who did not have a substance use disorde (7.0 percent), according to a 2003 report from the Substanc Abuse and Mental Health Services Administratio (SAMHSA).

- 37% of alcohol abusers and 53% of drug abusers also have a least one serious mental illness.

Additionally, The National Institute of Mental Health has sponsore two of the research studies on the groups most commonly affected b substance abuse.

- 10 million Americans are affected by a dual-diagnosis disorde each year.

- 56% of individuals with a bipolar disorder (Manic depressiv illness) abuse substances

- 47% of individuals with a schizophrenic disorder abus substances

- 32% of individuals with a mood disorder other than bipola abuse substances

- 27% of individuals with an anxiety disorder abuse substances.'

These large percentages look very different from an overall 15% o substance abuse disorders in the general population.

A central question about dual diagnosis is which came fist – th substance abuse or the psychiatric disorder? Research has shown tha it can go either way.. Often the psychiatric problem develops first. Ir an attempt to feel calmer, more energized and alert, or more joyful, a person with emotional problems may use drugs or drink to sel medicate. Frequent self-medication may eventually lead to a dependency on alcohol or drugs. If it does, the person then suffers from not just one problem, but two. In adolescents, however, drug or alcohol abuse may merge and continue into adulthood, which may ontribute to the development of emotional difficulties or psychiatric isorders.

n other cases, alcohol or drug dependency is the primary condition. A erson whose substance abuse problem has become severe may evelop symptoms of a psychiatric disorder including episodes of epression, anger, hallucinations, or suicide attempts. n terms of treatment for dual diagnosis, people have asked which iagnosis should be treated first. It is often difficult to separate what ymptoms belong to which diagnosis. Since many symptoms of ubstance abuse mimic or mask other psychiatric conditions, the erson must go through withdrawal from alcohol and/or other drugs efore the clinician can accurately assess whether there is a psychiatric roblem also.

That being said, research has concluded that both problems should be reated simultaneously or in an integrated fashion. For any substance abuser, however, the first step in treatment must be detoxification -- a eriod of time during which the body is allowed to cleanse itself of lcohol or drugs. For opioid addiction, it may be best to get the ddicted patient stabilized on methadone so that the withdrawal and raving aspects can be suspended. Some persons with co-existing sychiatric problems will need mental health evaluation and treatment o get through detoxification or stabilization.

Psychiatric Services Within A Substance Abuse Health Care Program

Addicted patients already in early in recovery are generally referred or assessment and stabilization of psychiatric symptoms. 70% of this population comes from the legal justice system. These patients meet the criteria for *Dual-Diagnosis*, i.e., having both an addiction and a psychiatric diagnosis. This is also referred to as *co-occurring disorders*. Drug addicts present with the same psychiatric conditions as the public at large, hence common problems tend to be prevalent among addicts too. Although women traditionally present with depression, men present with problems that are more consistent with aggression and impulsivity. It is vital to establish rapport with these patients, since the psychiatrist may be their first contact with a mental health professional.

Addicts tend to have a complicated presentation, mostly due to the involvement with law agencies, dependency court, and unemploymen Many are recently released from jail and have lost all of thei possessions. Not only do they have to deal with mental illness, bu also the realities of a complex legal and social structure that is ver demanding of their time and emotions. Some patients are als homeless or staying in temporary housing. Indeed, their stress level i high, sleep is often disrupted, and they may not have access to an services let alone psychiatric treatment.

After an initial psychiatric work-up, a list of symptoms is generate with the help and participation of the patient, which upon thei resolution, become the criteria for discharge. Patients are encourage to focus on their symptoms and discomfort, rather than diagnosis.

In an average year, 500 to 750 patients receive psychiatri evaluation/treatment. Although the patients are told the program i voluntary, the majority finishes the 3-4 months course witl improvement and achieves psychiatric stability. These patients ar then referred preferably to a primary-care physician for continued medical care.

The Mood Disorders---Depression

The term *Mood Disorders* covers up to 70-75% of all psychiatri presentations. This includes all types of depression, bipolar disorde and the related anxiety and psychosis. They cause major financia burden on the economy due to loss of productivity, lower immunity and predisposition to health problems. Suicide and hospital stays cos huge sums of money. The focus nowadays is to get these patients wel fast and achieve remission.

The most common diagnosis is Major Depression, with or withou psychotic features.

Although the symptoms and presentation varies for different individuals, lack of pleasure, sad mood, and lack of motivation top the list. Suicidal ideation may be present with or without history of attempts. Although there is a notion that addicts "treat themselves" with street drugs, it is not clear whether addicts carry a diagnosis of major depression more than the general population. Typically addicts carry the burden of financial, legal and custody problems, more than the average person. It may be argued that they are more disposed to "situational depression" given how chaotic their lives may be. It is also true that once an addict stops using stimulants, e.g. amphetamines, it seems that they are more predisposed to weight gain, sleep problems, poor concentration and attention. These cluster of symptoms are commonly referred to as vegetative symptoms of depression.

It seems that major depression rarely exists in a pure form. Anxiety and related disorders are seen up to 90% of the cases. There is a debate whether these co-existing conditions are a cause of, a result of, or just a related condition to depression. Common one is agoraphobia, generalized anxiety disorder, panic attacks and post-traumatic stress disorder.

In the last decade, there has been more emphasis on bipolar (manic-depressive) disorder, and the fact that a patient can present with psychosis as part of their manic-hypomanic states. Good psychiatric skills are needed to decide what cause of psychosis is being faced with. Bipolar disorder encompasses a wide variety of symptoms, with life-long disabilities. Symptoms can be treated in an outpatient setting, but more serious presentations may require hospitalizations and even residential placements.

Mania is the extreme and dramatic presentation of this disorder. Laymen can recognize the severity of this condition due to erratic and dangerous actions these patients embark on. Manic patients require no or limited sleep, are hypersexual, spend money foolishly and tend to make long distance call at odd hours. They may disrobe, expose themselves, are loud with pressured speech. They can be angry, irritable and even grandiose and psychotic. They may think they are God, a president or other important figures. Unfortunately such a presentation can be caused by stimulant drugs and even steroids, hence the difficulty in initial diagnosis.

Treatment

Antidepressants, known as SSRI's for the their action on Serotonin are widely prescribed in this population. Common ones are Prozac, Zoloft, Paxil, Celexa and Lexapro. Not only they improve symptoms of depression, but anxiety, a very common associate of depression also improves. Typically addicts complain of anxiety and restlessness. Given the SSRI's safety records as compared to tricyclic (traditional antidepressants), they are by far the most common prescribed psychotropic medicine.

The most common side effects from SSRI's come from their effect on increase Serotonin in the nervous system in general. Weight gain, gastro-intestinal pain, tops the list of common side effects. They may also affect sleep, appetite and weight. Sexual side effects are as high as 20-25%, but patients usually do not complain about them. Decrease libido, and delayed or no ejaculation are typical in men, and to a lesser degree in women.

Suicidal behavior and completed suicide have been the focus of media and political groups. Recent data give conflicting reports as to the prevalence of this problem, but it has been adopted by the psychiatric community as a required element of the psychiatric evaluation. Children, adolescents and adults are all at risk.

Other antidepressants are gaining market share due to effectiveness, different side effect profile, and some without the sexual side effects and weight gain. Wellbutrin, also sold as Zyban for smoke cessation, is unique because of its action on norepinephrine and to less extent on dopamine. It causes no sexual, weight gain side effects, but is a powerful activating agent that can cause insomnia and agitation.

Dual action antidepressants like Effexor and Cymbalta are becoming replacement agents if SSRI's failed to achieve improvement (remission). Remeron causes weight gain and sedation.

Anxiety Disorders

Generalized anxiety disorder can be difficult to diagnose due to its prevalence and co-existence with other psychiatric conditions. Rapid heart beat, sweaty palms, and feeling of losing one's mind and losing control are very common. Its is common for non-Caucasians to experience anxiety as somatic complaints, e.g. headaches, backaches, stomachache, and even painful menses. Typically, an internist is able to rule physical causes of such presentations. Its is important to know how your patient thinks of anxiety since it is so variable.

PTSD (post-traumatic stress disorder) became widely known as a result of traumatic exposure during the Vietnam War, and later subsequent wars. Currently it is used to describe the after effects of any exposure to a serious trauma, including child abuse and sexual exploitation. The hallmark of this condition is hyper arousal, i.e., an increase symptoms anxiety, feelings of worthlessness and has pending doom. Depression is almost always present, but can be masked by frank anxiety and restless. Other anxiety disorders can also present in the same individual. Adults and children respond best to antidepressants in combination with support, group and individual therapy.

Obsessive-compulsive disorder is best described by "As good as it gets" movie where the actor has a need to repeat thoughts and actions to help control anxiety and a sense of loss of control. This condition is underreported due to the embarrassment of the patient, but usually admitted to upon inquiry. Depression can result from this condition due to its limiting and isolating results, but minor forms exists in successful and well-know individuals. Medication and behavioral techniques alone are equally effective, but best results are achieved when combined.

Benzodiazepines, like Ativan, Klonopin, Xanax, Valium and Librium are very effective anti-anxiety agents for the short-term treatment of the these disorders. Their main drawback is their addiction potential, hence there are inappropriate for long-term use. They have very limited side effects; hence they are superior to all other psychotropic medications. Infrequent use is the most beneficial way to treat occasional anxiety.

Psychotic Disorders

Psychosis is a very common presentation in this population. This ma include paranoid ideation, delusions and even frank hallucinatior Patients may not understand the seriousness of psychosis, and th evaluator has to ask specific questions about hearing voices, seein things, confusion, and thinking problems. If anger and impulsivit compound psychosis, disastourous results may affect such patients fo the rest of their lives. In most situations, hallucinations requir immediate if not urgent evaluation and intervention.

Psychosis is commonly seen with depression, although it can presen itself as "drug induced" psychosis, which improves fast. Visua hallucinations are more common with drug induced psychosis an mania, and auditory hallucinations are more common in schizophrenia Only 1-2% of this population is truly schizophrenic, and requires long term care and sometimes institutionalization. Although there are different forms of schizophrenia, for practical purposes and treatment there are grouped together as one major diagnosis category. Typically schizophrenic are treated by department of mental health due to the chronic nature of this disease.

Typical antipsychotics, like Haldol, Navane and Stelazine are rarely used nowadays due to their long-term side effects. Atypical or newei antipsychoticts have less side effect profile, are better tolerated, hence compliance is better. Not only psychosis improves, but depression, tc some extent, also gets better with these newer agents. There are six agents approved for use in this country, and include Clozaril, Zyprexa Seroquel, Geodon, Abilify and Risperdal.

Polypharmacy is a term used when more than two or three psychiatric medications are used. Apart from cost, added intolerable side effects, drug interactions and even masking of some of the symptoms may occur. Rarely, antidepressants do the job alone; hence a sleep aid is introduced. Psychosis requires the use of antipsychotic meds. I ipolar disorder is suspected, then mood stabilizers are used. It is ommon to see chronic patients on 3-4 psychotropic medications.

dult ADHD, although it has its roots in early childhood, is a rather ommon (10-15%) presentation in amphetamine abusers/addicts. mphetamines, like the stimulants physicians use for the treatment of nis disorder, help improve attention, focus, memory and a general eeling of well-being. With treatment, patients are more productive, inish projects and their organizational skills improve. In children, the nost prescribed medication is Ritalin. Although it is not an mphetamine, its stimulant action is very similar to amphetamine. Due o its addiction potential, its use in addicts is somewhat controversial.)exedrine and Adderall are amphetamine-based products; hence their se should be closely monitored. Non-stimulant medications are trattera and Wellbutrin which are alternatives in addicts. All of these nedications can curb the appetite and cause weight loss and insomnia.

ersonality disorders, also know as character disorders, are common mong this population. Sometimes these disorders are referred to as 'Axis II" diagnosis, referring to the DSM IV manual. Although it is ard to treat these disorders (e.g. antisocial and borderline), it is mportant to treat the accompanying symptoms of depression, anxiety, anic, obsessive-compulsive, and sleep problems. Treating these ymptoms improves the odds for these patients to stay clean, and rely ess on street drugs. Acting-out is common with this diagnosis, and he treating physician or therapist should be careful in preventing these atients from accusing them of improper or unprofessional conduct. They seem to always complain about their lives, and how the system nd provider are not helping them.

References

Regier, D. A., Farmer, M. E., Rae, D. S., et al., Comorbidity of mental disorders with alcohol and other drug abuse, JAMA 264(19):2511-2518 (1990).
Drake, R. E., Essock, S. M., Shaner, A., Carey, K. B., Minkoff, K., Kola, L., Lynde, D.,

Osher, F. C., Clark, R. E., & Richards, L. (2001). Implementing dual diagnosis services for clients with severe mental illness. *Psychiatric Services, 52,* 469-476.

Dual Diagnosis-The Problem (2005) from http://alcoholism.about.com/cs/dual/a/aa981209.htm

Foundations Associates (2004) from http://www.dualdiagnosis.org/index.php?id=9

Mueser, K. T., Bellack, A. S., & Blanchard, J. J. (1992) Comorbidity of schizophrenia and substance abuse: Implications for treatment. *Journal of Consulting and Clinical Psychology, 60,* 845-856.Nolen-Hoeksema, S. (2004). *Abnormal psychology.* (3rd ed.). New York: McGraw Hill.

Phillips, P., & Labrow, J. (2004). *Understanding dual diagnosis.* from http://www.mind.org.uk/Information/Booklets/Understanding/Understanding+dual+diagnosis.htm

Bridget F. Grant; Frederick S. Stinson; Deborah A. Dawson; S Patricia Chou; Mary C. Dufour; Wilson Compton; Roger P. Pickering Kenneth Kaplan. Prevalence and Co-occurrence of Substance Use Disorders and Independent Mood and Anxiety Disorders: Results From the National Epidemiologic Survey on Alcohol and Related Conditions. Arch Gen Psychiatry, Aug 2004; 61: 807 - 816.

Chapter 7

Methadone and Pregnancy

Deborah Stephenson, M.D.

Opioid Addiction in Pregnancy

Opioid addiction puts a woman, her pregnancy and her baby at increased risk of a negative outcome. Compared to a non-opioid addicted woman, there is a 3-7 times higher rate of stillbirth, fetal growth retardation (low birth weight and small head circumference), prematurity and neonatal mortality among women who use heroin while pregnant.

The lifestyle associated with drug use often interferes with a woman's ability to have a nutritious diet, to live in a safe and sober environment and to participate in prenatal care. Using drugs by injection puts the pregnant woman and her baby at risk of infection from contamination by bacteria in the drug/cut or by bacteria that live on the skin. If needles are shared with other persons, she is also at risk of acquiring blood borne diseases. Cleaning a shared needle with bleach may reduce the transmission of HIV infection, however it is not effective at preventing transmission of Hepatitis B and C.

Abrupt cessation of opioid use produces a constellation of effects that are dangerous for a pregnancy and a fetus. Withdrawal causes muscles to be overly active; the uterus is a muscle, so this can result in premature labor and/or delivery. Babies who are premature and/c small at birth are at much higher risk of infection, breathing, cardia and feeding problems and SIDS (Sudden Infant Death Syndrome When the body has become used to having opioids around constantly sudden cessation results in a whole cascade of neuro-hormona activity. The increased activity of the nervous system and stres hormone system creates an adverse in utero environment, which ca slow fetal growth or result in fetal death.

Medical Management of Pregnant Women with Opioid Addiction

In view of the medical risks posed by opioid addiction durin; pregnancy, prompt and effective medical treatment is needec Methadone Maintenance Treatment is the standard of care (in othe words, the treatment of choice) for any opioid addicted pregnan woman. Attempting to wean a pregnant woman off of an opioid i medically contraindicated.

In Santa Clara County opioid addicted pregnant women seekin; methadone treatment are admitted the day they call or the nex business day. Women who are incarcerated in Santa Clara County an found to be pregnant and opioid dependent are started on methadon maintenance while in jail and referred to the Perinatal Substanc Abuse Program and Central Valley Methadone Clinic upon discharge.

Eligibility criteria for admission to methadone maintenance are o necessity more lenient for pregnant women. Under Californi Regulations, any pregnant woman, with a history of opioid addiction who is currently physically dependent on an opioid, is eligible fo methadone maintenance treatment regardless of the duration o dependence.

Federal Regulations take it a step further. In recognition of the higl risk of relapse associated with a history of opioid addiction, Federa Regulations allow admission of any pregnant woman who is currentl physically dependent on opioids OR who has a history of dependence

nd is at risk of relapse even if she is not currently physically
ependent

nformed Consent for the Use of Methadone in Pregnancy

/Iany pregnant women are anxious about taking medication during
·regnancy. They feel particularly guilty about taking methadone
·ecause it makes them feel better, and they are worried that the
nedication will harm the baby. In addition, they do not want the baby
o experience methadone withdrawal at birth. Sometimes the situation
s complicated by a significant other, extended family member or
`riend who does not know the woman is on methadone or may not
:now that the woman has a history of opioid addiction at all or that she
vas using during the pregnancy. The woman is terrified that the
letails will become known at the time of delivery, either because
;omeone observes her taking her methadone dose or because the baby
las to stay in the hospital longer for observation or treatment of
leonatal abstinence.

t is vitally important for a pregnant woman being advised to start
nethadone maintenance to understand the benefits and risks of this
reatment and to be able to discuss her concerns with the prescribing
·hysician. Often multiple discussions are necessary over the course of
he pregnancy to provide reassurance regarding the safety of
nethadone during pregnancy and the necessity of a therapeutic dose to
:nsure the best possible outcome for mother and baby.

Methadone Maintenance Treatment is voluntary and is only started
after the patient gives written informed consent. Women are also
asked to provide written consent for the Methadone Physician to
coordinate with the Prenatal Care Provider and Pediatrician. Ongoing
·work with a counselor helps the woman to plan for delivery and to
deal with family and friends around this issue.

·Pregnant women are also afraid that taking methadone will increase
the chances that the baby will be taken by CPS at birth. This is most
unfortunate because a therapeutic dose of methadone and participation
in a treatment program vastly increases the chance that a woman will
be drug-free at delivery and able to take care of herself and a baby.

Polysubstance Abuse During Pregnancy

Polysubstance use is a common problem among pregnant wome
being admitted to methadone maintenance. Use of non-opioid drug
poses risks to a pregnant woman and her baby and may compromis
the efficacy of methadone treatment. Many patients will not voluntee
that they are using drugs other than opioids. It is important to as
directly, comprehensively and neutrally about all the various drugs an
to provide the level of treatment necessary to support cessation an
sustained abstinence from all drugs.

Treatment Goals During Pregnancy

Many of the treatment goals during pregnancy are the same as thos
for any patient on methadone maintenance as discussed elsewhere i
this document. These include: to fully suppress symptoms o
withdrawal between doses of methadone, to eliminate drug hunge
(unwanted thoughts about using or urges to use), to normaliz
physiologic functions disrupted by drug use, to block the effects o
illicit opioid use, to support sustained abstinence and participation in a
recovery program and to decrease risky behaviors.

Additional goals during pregnancy include: to increase participatior
in prenatal care, to improve maternal nutrition, to reduce obstetrica
complications, to minimize fetal drug exposure, to establish a
sustainable abstinence, to ensure a safe and stable living environmen
and to improve parenting skills.

Early and ongoing evaluation of each woman's situation is vital. This
evaluation can then be used to determine the intensity of treatmen
necessary to adequately address the combination of life problems that
could stand in the way of recovery. It may not be possible for a
woman to fulfill these treatment goals before delivery in an outpatien
setting.

Perinatal Drug Treatment

erinatal Drug Treatment Programs are designed to address gistical barriers and often include supports like onsite childcare, ansportation to and from program and onsite court approved arenting classes. Perinatal programs often include a more prominent edical component to address the numerous health issues associated ith addiction. The medical piece would include screening and eferrals at admission (medical, dental, public health nursing), weekly rine drug testing, regular visits with the physician at the methadone linic and coordination between the methadone physician and Prenatal are Providers and Pediatricians.

Medical Management of Methadone Maintenance During Pregnancy

he principles of induction described earlier in this document apply to regnant women. Because of the unique risks posed by untreated vithdrawal during pregnancy, a pregnant patient may be asked to emain onsite for observation longer on the first day or to return to the rogram later in the day for evaluation. Either of these will allow the dmitting physician to assess the patient when the medication is eaking in her system.

f symptoms of withdrawal persist, an additional dose can be given on he first day of treatment. Early in treatment, a pregnant patient may neet with the methadone doctor daily to every few days to assess the nethadone dose. Promptly and safely stabilizing the methadone dose s vital. Withdrawal needs to be completely suppressed to minimize isk to the fetus. The dose must be sufficient to support complete ibstinence. Sedation must be avoided as it results in fetal sedation, vhich could result in a newborn that has low blood pressure, low heart ate and respiratory suppression.

After the initial stabilization phase, a pregnant patient will meet with he methadone physician every 2-4 weeks depending on the severity of er addiction and complexity of her other medical problems. California Regulations require at least one methadone physician visit er month. At these follow-up visits, the methadone physician verifies hat the patient is participating in prenatal care, reassesses the adequacy and appropriateness of the methadone dose, reviews the urine drug test results and inquires about any drug use including use c opioid drugs and other illicit drugs (stimulants, THC, PCP, etc) an use of alcohol and cigarettes.

The methadone physician provides information regarding the risk associated with the use of drugs during pregnancy and works with th patient to address ongoing use of any of these substances and t identify strategies to allow and support cessation and abstinence.

Patients who continue to use will be strongly encouraged to enter residential treatment program; the methadone physician will also ale the prenatal care provider. Coordination with the prenatal car provider helps to assure that prompt and appropriate medica intervention is provided in the event of a drug-related complicatior allows the prenatal care provider to reinforce the recommendation t enter residential treatment and to provide medical counsel regardin the risks of drug use in pregnancy.

During follow up visits the methadone physician provides medica counsel regarding the importance of prenatal care, good nutrition preventive health care (tetanus boosters, HIV and Hepatitis testing) breastfeeding while on methadone, pain control during and afte delivery, contraception, post-partum depression.

The Effects of Pregnancy on Methadone Metabolism

Often a pregnant woman's dose needs to be adjusted as her pregnancy progresses. Pregnancy increases a woman's blood volume and may increase the rate at which methadone is broken down to its inactive metabolite. These changes mean that the woman's methadone bloo level often fall as her pregnancy progresses, resulting in emergence o symptoms of withdrawal. The methadone dose must be increased ir this situation, until symptoms of withdrawal are completely suppressed.

The most commonly seen pattern is that the methadone dose needs tc increase during the first and the third trimesters and remains fairly onstant during the second trimester. In some women, this can be ramatic, with the methadone dose doubling over the course of the regnancy. In these patients, measuring the methadone blood level onfirms that the level falls dramatically during the pregnancy and ses again after delivery. These patients need the dose decreased after elivery to prevent sedation. Some pregnant women cannot be tabilized on one dose a day and must take a morning and evening ose of methadone to prevent emergence of symptoms of withdrawal.

Iethadone Maintenance Alone is Insufficient to Treat Opioid ddiction in Pregnancy

n addition to the medical issues surrounding heroin dependence, the eroin-addicted patient frequently comes from a severely disordered amily. The intensity of chaos and dysfunction seen with heroin ddiction surpasses that associated with other substances. There is •ften brokenness that encompasses every aspect of the woman's life. •regnancy in this setting complicates the problem.

;ome of the problems include: homelessness, inadequate resources or food/clothes/other basic needs, hazards in the home environment unsafe area, uncontained dogs, lack of hot water, rats, toxic :hemicals), domestic violence, drug using family or friends in the iome, lack of parenting skills, school-aged children in the home who ire not enrolled in school, involvement with criminal justice, nvolvement with social services, no high school diploma, little or no vocational skills/training, lack of access to medical/dental care, intreated chronic/acute medical/dental problems, poor nutrition, ;evered relationships with healthy/sober family/friends.

•erhaps the most critical issue when treating the heroin-addicted •regnant patient is to understand that unless multiple issues are iddressed simultaneously, treatment is not likely to be successful. It is iecessary to assess thoroughly and repeatedly in an effort to inderstand the patient's life situation, so that a comprehensive plan :an be formulated which allows the patient to achieve abstinence. 3arriers to participating in treatment must be identified and dealt with.

Participation in individual and group counseling at the program is a critical part of treatment. Perinatal programs often offer classes abou addiction, recovery, pregnancy, parenting, healthy relationships an life-skills. Mommy and Me programs teach women how to care fc and play with their infants and young children. Parent Support Group encourage women to share their parenting challenges and concerr and to learn from one another under the guidance of a knowledgeabl staff person.

The majority of women who are on methadone maintenance com from very troubled family situations and received inadequate parentin themselves, so need ongoing coaching, modeling and support. Man Perinatal Programs have health educators on staff to teach wome about issues such as normal child development, dental hygiene, how t feed a child, how and when to toilet train, etc. Referral to Publi Health Nursing may also be helpful, so that a nurse can go out to th house to assess and assist.

In Utero Methadone Exposure and the Neonatal Abstinenc Syndrome

Fetal methadone exposure is known to be safer than fetal heroi exposure or fetal opioid withdrawal. Methadone has been used an studied for 40 years. As NIDA states, "Research has demonstrate that the effects of in utero exposure to methadone are relativel benign." There are no known birth defects associated with its us during pregnancy. Methadone Maintenance of the opioid dependen woman increases the likelihood that the mother will participate i prenatal care and that the baby will be born at term.

Methadone exposed babies generally have lower birth weights/smalle head circumferences than non-opioid exposed babies, but higher birtl weights/larger head circumference than heroin exposed babies. While methadone exposed babies tend to have lower birth weights than non exposed babies, the birth weights are within the normal range fo newborns.

xposure to any opioid in utero (heroin or methadone) increases the ate of SIDS by 3-4 times that seen in the general population. 1ethadone exposed neonates may have an increased platelet count tarting in the first or second month of life, which may persist for 6-10 1onths; no adverse outcomes have been described as a result of this. 'inally in utero methadone exposure may elevate the level of two nyroid hormones (T3 and T4) during the first week of life. I have not een able to find anything in the literature indicating that this elevation s clinically problematic.

A number of studies have looked at the long-term effects of in utero nethadone exposure. The data indicate that there are no uniform long-erm effects of methadone maintenance treatment during pregnancy. nfants exposed to methadone in utero have normal physical and nental development as children. Environmental factors, family haracteristics and functioning play a significant role in a child's levelopment. It should be noted that many opioid dependent patients moke cigarettes. Exposure to cigarettes in utero and after birth ncreases the risks of SIDS (sudden infant death syndrome or crib eath), ADHD and learning disorders.

Methadone exposed babies may experience symptoms of methadone vithdrawal after birth. Symptoms may include: tremors, hyperactive tartle reflex, irritability, high-pitched cry, poor feeding, vomiting, liarrhea, hyper-tonicity (stiff muscles), sneezing, sweating. Untreated vithdrawal may progress to seizures and death. This constellation of ymptoms in an opioid exposed baby is known as the Neonatal Abstinence Syndrome (NAS).

According to some published literature, the frequency of NAS may be is high as 60-80% of methadone-exposed babies. Two more recent tudies (2002 and 2005) found a NAS rate of 46%. NAS begins within the first 14 days of life. It is usually treated with a morphine or nethadone solution given by mouth or by feeding tube. Medical evaluation and treatment of suspected NAS is critical, because untreated NAS may lead to neonatal seizures or death. The duration of treatment is days to months. An experienced physician and facility safely and easily manage NAS.

The severity of withdrawal in the neonatal period does not impact IQ scores later in life. Methadone exposed infants are within the normal range of development and do not differ in cognitive function from non-exposed infants matched for socio-demographic, biological and health factors.

There is not a straightforward relationship between a pregnant woman's methadone dose and the baby's risk of NAS. "Higher" doses of methadone do not increase the risk of NAS but do increase the likelihood of the mother achieving abstinence. The risk of NAS appears to be related to the mother's and the baby's methadone blood level at delivery and how quickly the baby's blood level drops off in the first 4 days of life. Babies appear to be at higher risk if the mother and baby had a low methadone blood level or if the baby's methadone blood level drops quickly. In my clinical experience, withdrawal is more likely if the pregnant woman is unstable, meaning she is using drugs (heroin or other) in addition to methadone. However, there has not been a study to evaluate the effects of non-opioid fetal drug exposure on the expression of NAS. In addition maternal withdrawal close to the time of delivery appears to increase the risk of neonatal withdrawal. It has been postulated that a twice a day dosing schedule which decreases the likelihood of maternal withdrawal may decrease the risk of NAS.

In my clinical experience, it is not uncommon for a stable methadone maintained woman with an average methadone dose (80-120 or higher) to have a baby with no symptoms of NAS or very mild symptoms, not progressing or requiring treatment. These babies are able to go home with their mother at day of life 3 provided the mother understands the necessity of bringing the baby in promptly should symptoms of withdrawal occur.

Toxicology Testing at Delivery

Drug screening at delivery is recommended for pregnant women with a history of addiction. The results provide information that may impact the medical management of the mother and child. Testing also provides documentation of the woman's status at delivery, which may ssist with decisions regarding the custody of the child. A positive rug-screening test at delivery (particularly a term and therefore nticipated delivery) is a red flag for a more serious addiction roblem. It may indicate that drug use is beyond the woman's ability ɔ control, meaning that a more intensive level of care is needed.

Pain Management

Labor, delivery and the post-partum period often involve significant mounts of pain. Opioid dependent persons are more sensitive to pain; his is a neurological reality. When taken once/day, methadone does ıot provide pain relief. Additional medications will be needed for pain nanagement. Untreated pain may trigger cravings or relapse in a ɔerson with a history of addiction. For mild pain, Acetaminophen or buprofen will often be adequate. For moderate to severe pain, short-ıcting opioids will be needed on top of the regular dose of methadone. 3ecause of higher tolerance to opioids, addicted patients often need loses at the upper end of the therapeutic range to experience pain elief. Discharge pain medications should be prescribed if pain is ınticipated (after C/S or traumatic vaginal delivery). Caution should ɔe used about the quantity of medication sent home and availability of efills. A few days supply with the availability of a refill or two on ipecified dates to cover the anticipated painful period may be ıdvisable. The prescribing physician will bring patients in for ɔvaluation if refills are requested beyond the anticipated period.

Breastfeeding While on Methadone Maintenance

Breastfeeding has many known advantages for mother and baby and should be encouraged provided there is no contraindication. Methadone is not a contraindication as negligible amounts of methadone are present in breast milk, not enough to affect the baby. Because of this, breastfeeding cannot be used to prevent or treat NAS. It is important that a woman be stable in recovery if she plans to breastfeed to avoid exposing the baby to drugs of abuse that may be passed in breast milk.

In addition the woman's HIV status and risk factors need to be evaluated. HIV is passed in breast milk, so mothers infected with HIV should not breast feed. It normally takes about 2 months from the time of HIV exposure for the infection to be detected by testing. Mother who have tested negative for HIV but who have recent risk factor must be counseled regarding the risk of transmission.

The mother's hepatitis B and C status must also be considered. Women need to be given information, so they can make an informed decision. Traditionally, hepatitis B infection was considered to be medical contraindication for breastfeeding. Hepatitis B virus i present in breast milk. Transmission from mother to child is most likely to occur as a result of the delivery process. When a mother has hepatitis B, the baby is treated at birth to decrease the risk of transmission. The baby is given the first vaccination of a three shot Hepatitis B series. The vaccination protects by stimulating the baby' immune system to make antibody that will attack the Hepatitis B virus. It takes time for the vaccine to work, so the baby is also given Hepatitis B immune globulin (HBIG). HBIG is ready-made antibody that can begin fighting hepatitis B virus immediately. These interventions decrease the risk of transmission via breast milk by about 95%. While Hepatitis C is not present in breast milk, it is present in blood. According to the CDC, a woman with Hepatitis C may breastfeed, but must discontinued, pump and discard in the event o nipple trauma until she has healed.

Other Post-Partum Concerns

The methadone physician meets with the patient after delivery to evaluate the methadone dose, screen for post-partum depression, discuss the risk of relapse, encourage ongoing participation in the program, and remind the patient to follow-up with the Ob/Gyn physician for post-partum care and contraception.

The methadone physician evaluates the appropriateness of the methadone dose fairly soon after delivery. Some women will experience sedation as their body returns to the non-pregnant state. This can happen quickly in some women and more slowly in others.

arly detection of sedation and dose adjustment is essential to nsure that the mother is able to care for her infant.

ost-partum depression in a woman with a history of addiction puts er at risk of relapse. It also may impair maternal-infant bonding, nterfere with parenting and rob a woman of the enjoyment associated vith caring for a new baby. Many depressed women do not recognize nat the symptoms they are experiencing are due to depression, so they nay not seek medical evaluation and treatment. Educating women efore delivery about post-partum depression may be helpful. Prompt iagnosis and treatment is essential.

he methadone physician and program counselors make an effort to tay in contact with women after delivery and encourage them to eturn to program as soon as reasonably possible. Caring for a new aby can be overwhelming and getting organized to get out of the ouse with the baby is challenging. However mothers in recovery are articularly vulnerable to relapse at this time, so the support of the reatment program is vital.

What About Methadone Withdrawal After Delivery?

Discontinuation of methadone treatment after delivery is medically ontraindicated because it almost inevitably results in relapse to daily llicit opioid use. As reported by Ball and Ross in 1991, the relapse ate is 80% within the first year of withdrawal. Methadone Maintenance Treatment is effective long-term medical treatment for he chronic disease of opioid addiction.

The post-partum period is a difficult time for any woman because of he intense demands of a newborn at a time when she is physically rying to recover from delivery. Women in general need increased upport during this time. It is a particularly bad time to withdraw the upport of a necessary and effective medication.

References

Ball, J.C. and Ross, A. (1994). The Effectiveness of Methadone Maintenance Treatment. New York: Springer-Verlag.

Jones, Carolyn W., MSN, RNC, NNP. (2004). Platelet Disorders. Newborn & Infant Nursing Reviews. 4(4):181-190.

Joseph, Herman, Stancliff, Sharon & John Langrod, (2000 Methadone Maintenance Treatment (MMT): A Review of Historica and Clinical Issues The Mount Sinai Journal of Medicine. 67(5,6):347 364.

Kaltenbach, Karol A. (1996). Exposure to Opiates: Behaviora Outcomes in Preschool and School-Age Children. NIDA Monograp 164:230-241.

Kaltenback, K & Finnegan, L.P. (1987). Perinatal and developmenta outcome of infants exposed to methadone in-utero. Neurotoxicc Treratol 9(4):311-3.

Kaltenbach, K & Finnegan, L.P. (1984). Developmental Outcome o Children Born to Methadone Maintained Women: a review o Longitudinal studies. Neurobehav Toxicol Teratol 6(4):271-5.

Kaltenbach, D.; Graziani, L.J. & Finnegan, L.P. (1979). Methadon Exposure In Utero; Developmental Status at One and Two Years o Age. Pharmacol Biochem Behav 11 Suppl:15-7.

Kaltenbach, K.A. & Finnegan, L.P. (1989). Prenatal Narcoti Exposure: Perinatal and Developmental Effects. Neurotoxicolog 10(3):597-604.

Lawrence, Ruth A., Lawrence, Robert M. (1999). Breastfeeding: A Guide for the Medical Professional. St. Louis, Missouri: Mosby.

McCarthy, John J., Leamon, Martin H., Parr, Michael S., Anania Barbara. (2005). High-Dose Methadone Maintenance in Pregnancy Maternal and Neonatal Outcomes. American Journal of Obstetrics and Gynecology. 193:606-610.

McCarthy, John J., Possey, B.L. (2000). Methadone Levels in Human Milk. Journal of Human Lactation. 16(2): 115-120.

rinciples of Addiction Medicine, third edition (2004). Chevy
'hase, Maryland: American Society of Addiction Medicine.

.osen, Tove S. & Johnson, Helen L. (1985). Long-Term Effects of
'renatal Methadone Maintenance. NIDA Monograph 59:73-83.

.andall, Stephen R. (1993). Improving Treatment for Drug-Exposed
nfants: Treatment Improvement Protocol (TIP) Series 5DHHS
'ublication No. (SMA) 93-2011.

'olton, Kimberly, Dietrich, Kim, Auinger, Peggy, Lanphear, Bruce &
Hornung, Richard. (2005). Exposure to Environmental Tobacco
.moke and Cognitive Abilities Among
J.S. Children and Adolescents. Environmental Health Perspectives
  13(1)

.ickler, Patrick, (1999). MERIT Award Research Helps Reveal Long-
erm and Developmental Impact of Dug Abuse. NIDA Notes 14(1):1-
..

Chapter 8

Myth, Misunderstanding & Stigma

Robert B. Kahn, Ph.D.

The continued hesitation by many to recognize addiction as a medical disease may be symptomatic of a societal ambivalence about the use of drugs. Many Americans regularly consume some psychoactive drugs including alcohol, cigarettes, and caffeine, as well as prescription medications - especially for anxiety and depression. Anti-anxiety medications alone, for example, accounted for $1 billion in expenditures in 1996 and an estimated 100 million prescriptions were written in 1999.

Understandably, few people can identify themselves with injection drug users and consequently there is little empathy or compassion for them. This dynamic is only one of several factors that can lead to myth and misunderstanding about opioid addiction and methadone treatment. Interestingly, this dynamic seems to lessen significantly for the use of alcohol or prescription drugs and, to some extent, with tobacco, marijuana, or even cocaine. Presumably, this is because more people are familiar with, and therefore can more easily identify with, these types of drug use, as they have become more of a social norm compared to injecting heroin.

Not uncommonly, people will sometimes jokingly admit that they "simply cannot live without that morning cup of coffee", but i seriously challenged, would probably deny any lack of control issue about their daily consumption. The long lines at popular coffee cafe seem eerily similar to street addicts in search of their "fix". Suc incongruities can blur the distinctions between use and abuse an perpetuate many of the myths and misunderstanding about addictio and addiction treatment and specifically about methadone treatmer for opioid addiction.

Understanding the "Addict"

The landscape of addiction has changed over the years. During th 1950' s the Traditional *Addict (TA),* emerged. The TA was usuall African American or Hispanic, poorly educated, and involved with th criminal justice system. Besides using heroin, marijuana and alcoho were also consumed. By the 1970's, the Addicted *Poly Drug Use (APU)* entered the picture, addicted to narcotics, but frequentl consuming hallucinogens and stimulants, as well. The APU include better-educated and more affluent Caucasians, as well as an increase i the numbers of women. The addict moved from the barrio and ghett to Main Street.

Clearly, no one is immune from drug addiction. Heroin addiction doe not discriminate nor does it show preference for any socio-cultura condition and yet in the minds of many, there is a stereotypical imag of what an addict typically looks like.

Understanding the Treatment

There is a plethora of medical and clinical research evidence tha methadone treatment not only saves lives, but millions of dollars ir health care and criminal justice costs as well. The medication itself i next to miraculous, given that it is orally administered, cross-toleran with some other narcotics, and provides relief for 24 hours or more.

all true, why conflict? The continuing controversy about methadone treatment is found both in the genesis of the medication and the disease of opioid addiction itself.

The public's first introduction to the "treatment" of narcotic addiction was the invention of heroin by the German Bayer Corporation in 1897. Heroin was touted as a cure for "Morphinism". Obviously, not long after heroin's initial legal use for the treatment of opiate addiction, the original "cure" became itself the problem.

In the United States, the first official "Treatment Plan" for narcotic dependency came during the early part of the twentieth century. Heavily weighted in favor of " law and order", it all but ignored health and safety". Between 1914 and 1938, approximately 25,000 physicians were arrested and 5,000 jailed for attempting to treat narcotic dependence. Thus, the stigma against both the opioid addicted patient and the treatment provider was established.

In 1937 during World War II, analgesics were in short supply in Germany. A major funding source of the Nazi regime had synthesized methadone and it became a major political and social issue impeding its widespread acceptance. The major funding source, I.G Farben Corporation, was also the one that later supplied Zyklon-B, used to exterminate millions. Eli Lilly introduced methadone into the United States in 1946, under the trade name "dolophine" (from the word "dolar" or pain). The choice of name and its similarity to Adolph Hitler lent credence to those believing it was developed to enslave, not treat.

Methadone treatment emerged in the U.S. as a pragmatic and cost effective approach compared to the devastating health and social consequences of opioid dependency. Prior to this, the U.S. unsuccessfully employed every intervention imaginable, including criminal incarceration, hospitalization, and intensive multidisciplinary inpatient medical and clinical therapies.

Following the 1965 work of Dr.'s Dole and Nyswander, articles about methadone from the then leading magazines led the public to falsely believe that a panacea for the eradication of narcotic addiction had been found. Drs. Dole and Nyswander would be the first to say tha methadone is not a cure but an invaluable assist in a narcoti dependent patient's recovery.

As recently as 1984, the United States Supreme Court denied veteran' benefits to alcoholics on the grounds that their condition is due t "*willful misconduct*". Vincent Dole, M.D. who, along with Mari Nyswander, M.D., pioneered methadone treatment, commented, "th ruling made explicit by the widespread prejudice against addicts.... i taken to logical limits, we would deny treatment to a skier with broken leg or a sunbather with skin cancer".

There are those that would believe methadone treatment actuall *creates addicts*. The criteria for substance dependence (addiction) a defined by the DSM IV includes a reference to the loss of control ove drug use and compulsive drug seeking/using behavior where thi behavior continues despite adverse physical, mental, legal, social, an occupational consequences. When an opioid addicted individual i stabilized on methadone, they no longer meet the diagnostic criteri for substance dependence.

Unfortunately, treatment or the lack thereof, is dictated by th perceptions held regarding opioid dependency per se, and only secondarily by the benefits of any particular treatment modality Today, even with the opportunities provided under Proposition 36 California Courts are reluctant to refer opioid dependent persons te methadone treatment, believing that "medicating" these patients is no a viable treatment option.

More than 210,000 patients are being treated in approximately 110(medically assisted treatment programs across the country. Methadon is but one component of these comprehensive medical and clinica treatment systems. These programs address the needs of their patients but as importantly, safeguard the general public as well

Addiction is a chronic and relapsing disorder, defying easy explanation or solutions.

he treatment of addictions, in the absence of scientific knowledge nd understanding, is reduced to a faith versus science debate. Believers" can't say enough about methadone treatment, while "non elievers" criticize its premise.

References

Brecher, Edward, M. and the Editors of Consumer Reports Magazine, The Consumer Union Reports on Licit and Illicit Drugs, 1972.

Drug Abuse Council, The Facts About Drug Abuse. 1980, The Free Press, New York.

Rajender, a., Mort J., Brandt, H. Psychotropic Medication Expenditures for Community-Dwelling Elderly Persons. May 2003, Psychiatric Services, Psychservices, psychiatryonline.org, Vol 54, No.5

Negroponte, Michel, "Methadonia". October 2005, HBO Special.

Dole, Vincent, "Implications of Methadone Maintenance for Theories of Narcotic Addiction", JAMA, 1988-Vol 260, No 20.

Addiction Treatment Forum, The Value of Addiction Treatment, Volume VIII#3, Summer 1999

Zarkin, G. New Study Finds Economic Benefit from Lifelong Methadone Treatment. November 16, 2006 News Release, Research Triangle Institute,

Altman, Heather, The Positive Effects of Psychotherapy on Methadone Maintenance Treatment, May 8, 2002, ALLPsych Journal.

Gerlach R. A Brief Overview On The Discovery of Methadone, 2004, V. Munster.

Hassin, Jeanette Hassin, Social Identity, Gender, and the Moral Self: The Intravenous Drug User and the Impact of AIDS, 1993, Doctoral dissertation, University of Arizona.

Zinberg, NE and RC Jacobson, The Natural History of "chipping". 1976, American Journal of Psychiatry, 133: 32-36.

Goldstein, A. Opioid Peptides (endorphins) in Pituitary and Brain. 1976, Science, 193:1081-1086.

Sackman, B., M.M. Sackman, and G.G. DeAngelis, Heroin Addiction as an Occupation; Traditional Addicted Polydrug Users. 1978, International Journal of Addictive Diseases 3, (2).

Sackman, Bertram S., A Comparison of Two Methadone Treatment Populations. 1976, an unpublished article.

Ausubel, David P., The Dole-Nyswander Treatment of Heroin Addiction, March 14, 1966, JAMA, Vol.195, No.11.

Kahn, R.B. 21-Day Outpatient Methadone Detoxification: An Evaluation, Part II. 1977-8, Drug Forum, Vol.6 (3).

Ball, J.C., and Ross, A. The Effectiveness of Methadone Maintenance Treatment. 1991, Springer-Verlag.

Weber, R.: Ledergerber, B.: et al. Cessation of Intravenous Drug Use Reduces Progression of HIV infection in HIV+ drug users. June 1990, Abstract of the Sixty International Conference on AIDS, San Francisco.

Ball, J.C.; Lange, R.W.; Myers, C.P.; and Friedman, S.R. Reducing The Risk of AIDS Through Methadone Maintenance Treatment. 1988, Journal of Health and Social Behavior, 29:214-226.

American Association for the Treatment of Opioid Dependence, www.aatod.org

My Story:

A Patient's Perspective

As is often the case for many addicts, I grew up in a troubled home and have often used my parents as scapegoats for my failures in life. My parents weren't really all that bad, they just didn't know how to express love and that lack of affection seemed to impact me more than it did my siblings. I was the youngest, living with an older brother and sister. Later, I learned of another sister who had been given up for adoption at birth.

My father was a sheriff whose job it was to investigate crime scenes, including homicide. My mother stayed at home to raise the children. However, she suffered from narcolepsy, a sleeping disease, which made this very difficult. She would take amphetamines to stay awake during the day and tranquilizers to sleep at night. I had been introduced to pot by my older sister so my mother's drugs provided a great opportunity for further experimentation. I was about twelve when I first smoked pot and by then my older brother had also joined law enforcement. The difficulty of hiding drugs in a home with two cops must have had something to do with slowing my progress.

When I was growing up, teachers told me I was bright and had "a lot of potential". I decided that I had had enough education and dropped out in the eleventh grade. One of my buddies whose mother was an alcoholic also dropped out so we left home and lived together. I remember we would take amphetamines that I was stealing from my mom and stayed up most of the nights wired and playing ping pong. Loyalty didn't have a high priority with me. I stole my friend girl friend and got her pregnant. I was fifteen years old at the time. It funny how some people react to responsibility. I ran and hid, or a least I tried. As I look back now it is clear to me that the reason began burglarizing homes was all about getting caught. For a ver scared fifteen-year-old boy, it was the easy way to avoid th responsibility of caring for a pregnant girlfriend, not to mention baby! I must have burglarized some sixty-plus homes before I finall got caught.

I soon got arrested again, this time for the mere possession of a ver small amount of pot--one roach! I was still on probation from my las episode with the law and the PO assigned to my case was a counselc who previously worked at the camp I had just left. He didn't like m and I didn't care for him much either. He told me that I had tw choices, either go to jail for a year or join the military. Since I hadn completed high school the Marine Corps was my only choice and the required a four-year enlistment.

It was early 1969, during the Viet Nam war. After about a year in th states I received orders for Vietnam. While in the military I stil managed to carry on in my old life style and could not put my pas behind me. While stationed in Okinawa, I was court marshaled for a combination of offenses, including possession of pot. They took all my stripes, fined me and restricted me to the base for several months However, I still had two and a half years remaining on my enlistmen and that gave me an opportunity to get back the stripes, a high schoo GED and an honorable discharge. It seemed my life had finally taken a turn in the right direction.

After leaving the military I began to fall back into my old behavio habits. I ran into some old friends whose drug use had escalated from pills to needles and that scared me. I started inhaling or snorting heroin but it wasn't long before I wanted to use the needle.

had a job when I first started but there are only a few jobs that ill support an addict's habit. The other problem is one's ability to unction while under the influence. Nodding is a dead give-away to hose who are savvy. I remember one day at the office my boss yelled ver the top of his partition for me to go home. I was too embarrassed to go home and that managed to wake me up so I lasted through the ay. I had held this job for about thirty months but realized that I had etter start looking for work elsewhere or risk getting fired.

started to replace my old habit with new ones. In place of heroin, I egan drinking alcohol and when I could scrounge some extra cash, nixed in a little cocaine. I became a full-blown alcoholic but nanaged to stay away from heroin, at least for a little while. In the Bay Area, I had no difficulty connecting with the patrons in local bars. One thing you learn about bars is that if you hang out long enough ou'll find whatever it is that you are looking for. In my case, it was eroin.

Before long I was back to my old habits and watching the familiar patterns reestablish themselves. I found another, job but it was not lose to home and I had no car. I began stealing money from my mployer. Then it was on to forging checks and stealing from department stores on my lunch breaks. Finally, I was arrested during ny lunch hour while stealing clothes from a department store.

My life was quickly deteriorating now. I found myself homeless and iving a meager existence in north Richmond. This was a new low point in my life, sleeping on an old mattress in a run-down apartment. remember the cockroaches, the tattered mattress on the floor, the 13 nch black and white TV with a coat hanger antenna and, most of all, he ever-present depression and shame. My days by now followed a consistent pattern. I would wake up, shower, dress and take off to nake money to support my habit. I would drive from one end of the Bay Area to the other and everyplace in between, looking for department stores to steal from.

t was only after the second time I was arrested that things took a turn for the better. It sure didn't feel like it at the time but once again I had experienced divine intervention in the form of a legal ultimatum. My choices were to get into an in-patient drug rehabilitation progran or go to jail. I just wasn't a jail kind of guy so I went with plan A After a brief stint in the hospital for detoxification I was accepted an transferred into a residential drug program.

After 18 months of living in a drug program I was deemed ready to g back to society and try again at becoming a productive member of th human race. While in the rehab program I was introduced to 12-step program philosophy and I managed to stick with it. A prerequisite fc a person to leave the inpatient program was to have gaine employment and established a support system, both of which I ha accomplished.

It was during a relationship that I slipped back into drug use. The warning signs were there, I stopped attending 12-step programs. wasn't drinking or using, but my mental state was on the verge o snapping despite the fact that I had held a job for seven years and ha advanced to a very responsible position in Regional Management. Thi time it started with my approaching one of the laborers where worked. I had asked around and knew this one particular guy wa dealing on the side so I took a huge risk and asked if he could get m some heroin. That eventually led to my changing jobs, it was just too risky now that other people at work knew of my habit. Following seven years at the same company I had managed to buy a home and save a little money. I bought the home with my current girlfriend and since the relationship was all but over, we had no alternative but to sel it.

I was so very tired of living my life like this. Spending years o rehabilitation only to see it all go down the drain and then to have to start all over again. Success followed by failure, followed by success failure and so on. I asked myself a thousand times if it would ever be any different. I had gone full circle and knew that I was but a step away from where I was at over a decade ago.

It was at that point that I made an appointment at the methadone clinic There is no doubt that this move gave me a new lease on life. It took

ome time for me to get back on my feet. It was not an easy ordeal
or me. I struggled for quite some time before I finally got back on my
eet. I left a job that had no future and found a position in a start up
ompany in the Silicon Valley. The company took off and shortly
nereafter I was promoted to a vice president position. I have no idea
what tomorrow will bring but for now I have a nice salary and live in a
ice neighborhood. I am married to wonderful woman who loves me
s much as I do her and I choose to simply enjoy what I have
ccomplished.

t has become clear to me that I am an incurable addict who cannot
xist without some form of medication. God knows that I tried every
venue available to me but they all eventually ended with my going
ack to drugs. I suppose that I could try again to live my life without
ome form of medication but based on my experiences, why would I
want to do that? I contracted hepatitis while sharing needles but with
he encouragement of the staff at the clinic and today's medications, I
ave managed to clear the virus.

FREQUENTLY ASKED QUESTIONS (FAQ) ABOUT METHADONE

s methadone addictive?

'hysical dependence and addiction are not the same. Methadone will ~roduce physical dependence (tolerance and withdrawal upon abrupt ~essation) but does not fuel the compulsive need for continued use ~espite adverse consequences, which is the cornerstone of addiction.

)o people who take methadone get high?

t was mentioned above that in order to experience the high, there ~nust be rapid uptake of the opiate in the brain. Methadone is taken up lowly so it does not produce the high. An excess of methadone ~esults in sedation, or somnolence called "nodding".

What are the benefits of being on methadone?   There are many ~easons. First, it avoids the dangers of transmitted viral diseases such ~s Hepatitis C and HIV. It avoids the bacterial infections, some of ~vhich can be life threatening, which result from the injection of ~mpure substances. Second, when a person is taking an appropriate, ~herapeutic dose, they can function normally. They can drive safely, ~hey can do virtually any kind of work (including executive positions), ~nd they can begin to reconstruct their lives their families and their ~elf-esteem.

How safe is methadone?

Methadone has very few side effects. It can cause a decrease in libido, ~vhich is common to all opiates. It can also cause some fluid retention, ~lsually early in treatment and spontaneously resolving. At very high ~loses, and in unusual circumstances methadone can cause ~rregularities of the heart beat. Methadone has now been prescribed on ~a daily basis to millions of patients for forty years and the adverse ~reactions are very few. Methadone does, however, interact with ~certain other prescribed medicine, such as some antibiotics and ~anticonvulsants. For this reason it is extremely important that patients taking methadone make that fact known to any other physicians or dentists who treat them.

Can you overdose on methadone?
Yes. All opiates share the liability that they depress the parts of the brain that control consciousness and respiration. If you take too much methadone, you become sleepy, and can lose consciousness. Ultimately the person becomes comatose, stops breathing and dies. Persons who are taking large amounts of heroin, or opium or morphine or methadone develop tolerance (see above)to these effects and are at less risk than persons who are naive to opiates
.

I've heard that methadone is bad for your liver. Is that true?
Absolutely not. There is no evidence that methadone in any way damages the liver. Many patients who are taking methadone have inflammation of the liver due to Hepatitis C infection. If methadone were bad for the liver we would have certainly seen evidence of that from the hundreds of methadone clinics around the world that are providing daily doses.

Do people have to stay on methadone for the rest of their lives?
Some do. As we discussed above, when patients want to stop taking methadone, they must be slowly tapered or they will have severe withdrawal symptoms which may cause them either to ask for their methadone dose to be increased, or worse, they will relapse to heroin use. There are people who are able to go through the taper and leave the program, which is encouraged by all responsible programs. These people are in the minority. Far more frequent is the experience that people attempt to taper and reach a point where they can no longer continue to lower the dose without enduring withdrawal symptoms and/or craving for heroin, their worst nightmare. They must then face the difficult decision that they may have to take methadone for the rest of their lives or risk relapse.

In a way, the situation is similar to that of a person with diabetes who has to take insulin for the rest of his life, or the person with hypertension who must take beta blockers for the rest of his life. These problems share common characteristics. They are chronic diseases that cannot really be cured. Persons with such diseases can, however, take medications to control the disease process. Other examples would be people with seizure disorders or with psychiatric problems who can live normal lives as long as they take their medicine.

Family members and friends will sometimes encourage people to stop taking methadone. "You're not using now so why don't you get off that stuff." They do not realize that the reason the person is no longer using is because of the methadone, and discontinuing therapy risks relapse. It would be similar to someone saying, "Now that your blood sugar is normal you should stop taking that insulin."

Selected Internet Sites

Below are some recommended websites for more information about methadone treatment and opioid addiction.

1. aatod.org. This is the American Association for the Treatment of Opioid Dependence, Inc. (AATOD).

2. asam.org. The American Society of Addiction Medicine (ASAM).

3. atforum.com. The Addiction Treatment Forum.

4. comproviders.com. The California Opioid Maintenance Providers (COMP).

5. drugpolicy.org. The Drug Policy Alliance.

6. nida.nih.gov. The National Institute of Drug Abuse (NIDA). Once on the website, go to the bottom right-hand side of the page and click on NIDA Notes Newsletter. When there, type in *methadone* on the search panel.

7. samhsa.gov. The Substance Abuse Mental Health Services Administration (SAMHSA). When on the site, go to the bottom of the page and click on Substance Abuse Treatment. Once on this page, find Medication Assisted Treatment and click to enter.

About the Authors

ALI ALKORAISHI, M.D.

Ali Alkoraishi, M.D. is the psychiatric consultant for the Santa Clara Valley Health & Hospital System Department of Alcohol & Drug Services. In this capacity, he provides treatment for system of care' dually diagnosed patients. He is also the Medical Director in Behavioral Health Services for the Catholic Charities agency. Dr. Alkoraishi is a psychiatric consultant on the use of the newest medications for the treatment of mental illness and dual diagnosis and has a specialty in pediatric psychiatry and the use of psychotropic medications in children. Dr. Alkoraishi has been teaching, consulting and practicing psychiatric medicine for twenty-five years.

DONALD R. AVOY, M.D.

Donald R. Avoy is a graduate of the University of Colorado and Stanford Medical School where he also did postdoctoral training in Internal Medicine and a fellowship in Hematology. Following that training he was in private practice and also served as Medical Director of the regional Red Cross Blood program in this area. He also spent several years as Medical Director of Syntex Diagnostic Division (SYVA). He has published many articles in scientific journals and is also the author of "Descent" a novel about heroin addiction.

Since 1997, Dr. Avoy has been with the Santa Clara Valley Health & Hospital System Department of Alcohol & Drug Services Addiction Medicine Division.

ROBERT GARNER

Robert Garner is the Director of the Santa Clara Valley Health & Hospital System, Department of Alcohol & Drug Services. For over thirty years, he has been the driving force behind the development of innovative and effective quality systems of care. As a recognized

ader in the substance abuse health care profession, Robert
Garner brings the most current research-based methods to efficiently
coordinate services and operate a large County Department. As the
Director, his Department was the first County in the State to develop a
managed and coordinated system of care for adult treatment. His
Department was also the first to fund a psychiatrist to provide for
dually diagnosed clients in the treatment system and the first County
to fund a network of transitional housing services to support clients in
recovery.

Recognizing that continuing education is key to maintaining a high
standard of care, Mr. Garner developed the Learning Institute and the
Research Institute focusing on implementing evidence – based best
practices in the County and bringing nationally renowned experts to
provide on-going training to the provider groups that comprise the
County's system of care. Robert Garner has brought forth the gold
standard for others to follow on how to blend high quality standards
into an integrated system of care that is strategic, evidence-based and
financially responsible

Robert Garner is also the Founding member and past President of the
California Association of County Drug and Alcohol Administrators
where he is currently the Chairman of the Youth Committee.

ROBERT B. KAHN, PH.D.

Robert B. Kahn is the President of the California Opioid Maintenance
Providers (COMP) and a Board Member of the American Association
for the Treatment of Opioid Dependence (AATOD). He holds a
Bachelor's, Masters, and Doctor of Philosophy Degree in Clinical-
Counseling Psychology. Dr Kahn is both a licensed Marriage &
Family Therapist and a Clinical Psychologist. He has taught at several
colleges and Universities and has written numerous articles on
behavioral health. He is also the author of the book, *To Your Health*,
offering insights into our biochemistry and psychology.

Since the late 1960's, Dr. Kahn has administered programs that treat
mental health and substance abusing patients. He first began treating

opioid dependency in 1969, and later helped to develop the first proprietary medically assisted (methadone) treatment in the Unite States. Dr. Kahn has administered and co-administered opioi treatment programs (OTP) throughout the country. In 2002, Dr. Kah sold his nationwide clinic system, then treating approximately 7,00 patients daily. He has served as a consultant to several States, as we as, the U.S., Polish, Bulgarian, and Hungarian Governments.

Dr. Kahn co-developed a toxicological and clinical laboratory continuing to provide the majority of toxicological screening fo Narcotic Treatment Programs (NTP) within the State of California a well as many outside of the state.

JUDITH MARTIN, M.D.

Judith Martin, M.D. is the Medical Director for the 14th Street Clinic She is also the Chair of the California Society of Addiction Medicin (CSAM) Committee for the Treatment of Opioid Dependence. D Martin is also the past President of CSAM.

SUMA SINGH, M.D.

Dr. Suma Singh completed primary medical training at Bosto University Medical School, and subspecialty training i Anesthesiology at Brigham & Women's Hospital/Harvard Medica School. During a Pain Management Fellowship at Stanford University Medical Center, she was introduced to Addiction Medicine while learning how to treat Chronic Pain in Addicted Patients at the Stanfor Hospital Inpatient Psychiatric Unit. Upon completion of he Fellowship, she began full-time clinical research in development o chronic pain medications with reduced abuse liability.

Dr. Singh began working with patients in Methadone Maintenance almost 10 years ago, while still engaged in full-time clinical research. Over the years, balance of patient care & clinical research shifted such that she currently works full-time as Medical Director for Departmen of Alcohol and Drug Services for Santa Clara Valley Health and Hospital System and provides teaching to VMC HHS physicians-in aining on the management of patients with addiction and chronic ain. She also intermittently provides clinical research consulting to ther research teams in these areas.

MARK STANFORD, PH.D.

Mark Stanford, Ph.D. is the Senior Manager of Medical and Clinical services for the Santa Clara Valley Health & Hospital System Department of Alcohol & Drug Services - Addiction Medicine and Therapy Division. He has direct clinical experience working in every modality of addictions treatment including inpatient, residential, day treatment, outpatient and opioid treatment programs. He has authored numerous materials in behavioral neuroscience including, *Foundations in Behavioral Pharmacology.*

Dr. Stanford is also a clinical research educator in the behavioral neurosciences. He has taught psychopharmacology throughout the Bay Area including a 20-year history with UC Berkeley Extension Department of Biological and Behavioral Sciences and Mathematics, and as a lecturer at Stanford University Department of Family and Community Medicine. He also teaches Treatment and Clinical Considerations of Substance Abuse Disorders for LCSW's, MFT's and Psychologists for their CEU licensing requirements.

DEBORAH STEPHENSON, M.D., MPH

Dr. Deborah Stephenson has been with the Santa Clara Valley Health & Hospital System Department of Alcohol & Drug Services since 1992 and has been providing medical management for the Perinatal Substance Abuse Program (including methadone maintained pregnant women) since 1993. She is certified in Addiction Medicine through the American Society of Addiction Medicine (ASAM) and Board Certified in Preventive Medicine/Public Health. She holds an MPH in Maternal and Child Health. Dr. Stephenson has been an active member of the California Society of Addiction Medicine (CSAM) Committee on Treatment of Opioid Dependence since its beginning in 1996. She was the primary Editor of the CSAM 2005 Guidelines for Physicians Working in California Opioid Treatment Programs.

JOAN ZWEBEN, PH.D.

Joan Ellen Zweben, Ph.D. is a clinical psychologist with over thirty five years' experience in treating addiction, and training treatment practitioners. These practitioners include peer counselors, social workers, marriage and family counselors, psychologists, probation officers, nurses and physicians. She has a broad based background in both alcoholism and drug dependence, and has experience with both residential and outpatient modalities. She has a long-standing commitment to building treatment resources through networking activities.

Dr. Zweben is the founder and Executive Director of The East Bay Community Recovery Project and The 14th Street Clinic & Medical Group and has steadily developed the medical and psychosocial services of these affiliated organizations. Her activities as an author, teacher, and consultant keep her informed of new developments in the field. She is the author of 3 books, over 55 articles or book chapters and editor of 15 monographs on treating addiction.

Dr. Zweben is a Clinical Professor of Psychiatry; University of California, San Francisco.

Made in the USA
San Bernardino, CA
25 July 2014